I will wait still 2 hours.

I will wait still 3 hours.

Etc.

I will wait still one day.

I will wait still 2 days.

I will wait still 3 days.

Etc.

Afer one hour or 2 hours or one day or 2 days passed by, ask yourself:

Do I feel the desire to drink alcohol?

No

In such a case you can continue with abstinence untill next time you feel the desire to drink alcohol.

Yes

In such a case you can make one more effort and one more time put untill later drinking alcohol again. Are you ready to make such an effort?

Yes

In this case you continue the abstinence.

No

In this case you are close to loose this time the battle with alcohol. This means you are not yet determined enough to continue the abstinence.

Try again later and never think when giving up drinking alcohol that it is for always. Always think it is for as long as possible.

Attention! Every time you give up alcohol you must get from your doctor drugs for the transition period between drinking alcohol and abstinence. Abrupt stop of drinking alcohol can be very dangerous for your health and even life.

***

Afternoon

* Repeat STOP (10 times every 30 min.)

* Say slowly every hour: sun, flower, seven, path, tee, run, yellow, apple, fish, rain, pen, water, smile, talk, life, sky.

* Dinner and half an hour break (you can sleep).

* Nice talk (no complaints) 30 min. When nobody to talk with, phone or internet conversation oral or written.

* Walk 15 min.

Most of the people who are addicted to alcohol do not know or do not want to know whether they are alcoholics. They believe untill late stages of the addiction they can more or less easily either control or stop drinking alcohol. But when they really try to stop drinking alcohol beverages they notice immediately that their organisms cannot do without alcohol. And this is the moment when alcohol addicted people all of a sudden discover with sorrow that this terrible thing happened to them! They have become alcoholics for the rest of their lives...

It is of course a very sad conclusion. But you should not dispair! There is a way to survive! It is possible to function normally without alcohol. It takes however several steps- the transition period.

Attention! If you notice that your body cannot do without alcohol when you stop drinking everyday, you should get specific drugs from your doctor to get over the transition period between drinking alcohol and abstinence.

After you made the transition period by means of specific drugs prescribed by your doctor for it, you can continue the self therapy like follows.

Week One

Day 1

Morning

* Repeat STOP (10 times every 30 min)

* Say slowly every hour: sun, flower, seven, path, tee, run, yellow, apple, fish, rain, pen, water, smile, talk, life, sky.

* Small physical excercise (10 min)

* Small breakfast.

* Nice talk (no complaints) 20 min. When nobody to talk with, phone or internet conversation oral or written.

* Walk 15 min.

* Every time the desire to drink alcohol comes back to you, imagine that you want to continue without alcohol only a little bit more. Never think that you will never ever drink alcohol again. Of course this would be great but for some people it is impossible to stand the idea, especially at the beginning of the therapy. But instead of breaking the abstinence right away, ALWAYS give yourself some time, even very short and say to yourself:

I will wait still one hour.

* Every time the desire to drink alcohol comes back to you, imagine that you want to continue without alcohol only a little bit more. Never think that you will never ever drink alcohol again. Of course this would be great but for some people it is impossible to stand the idea, especially at the beginning of the therapy. But instead of breaking the abstinence right away, ALWAYS give yourself some time, even very short and say to yourself:

I will wait still one hour.

I will wait still 2 hours.

I will wait still 3 hours.

Etc.

I will wait still one day.

I will wait still 2 days.

I will wait still 3 days.

Etc.

Afer one hour or 2 hours or one day or 2 days passed by, ask yourself:

Do I feel the desire to drink alcohol?

No

In such a case you can continue with abstinence untill next time you feel the desire to drink alcohol.

Yes

In such a case you can make one more effort and one more time put untill later drinking alcohol again. Are you ready to make such an effort?

Yes

In this case you continue the abstinence.

No

In this case you are close to loose this time the battle with alcohol. This means you are not yet determined enough to continue the abstinence.

Try again later and never think when giving up drinking alcohol that it is for always. Always think it is for as long as possible.

Attention! Every time you give up alcohol you must get from your doctor drugs for the transition period between drinking alcohol and abstinence. Abrupt stop of drinking alcohol can be very dangerous for your health and even life.

***

Evening

- Repeat STOP (10 times every 30 min.)

- Say slowly every hour: sun, flower, seven, path, tee, run, yellow, apple, fish, rain, pen, water, smile, talk, life, sky.
- Small supper.
- Nice talk (no complaints) 20 min. When nobody to talk with, phone or internet conversation oral or written.
- Walk 15 min.
- Every time the desire to drink alcohol comes back to you, imagine that you want to continue without alcohol only a little bit more. Never think that you will never ever drink alcohol again. Of course this would be great but for some people it is impossible to stand the idea, especially at the beginning of the therapy. But instead of breaking the abstinence right away, ALWAYS give yourself some time, even very short and say to yourself:

  I will wait still one hour.

  I will wait still 2 hours.

  I will wait still 3 hours.

  Etc.

  I will wait still one day.

  I will wait still 2 days.

  I will wait still 3 days.

  Etc.

Afer one hour or 2 hours or one day or 2 days passed by, ask yourself:

Do I feel the desire to drink alcohol?

No

In such a case you can continue with abstinence untill next time you feel the desire to drink alcohol.

Yes

In such a case you can make one more effort and one more time put untill later drinking alcohol again. Are you ready to make such an effort?

Yes

In this case you continue the abstinence.

No

In this case you are close to loose this time the battle with alcohol. This means you are not yet determined enough to continue the abstinence. Try again later and never think when giving up drinking alcohol that it is for always. Always think it is for as long as possible.

Attention! Every time you give up alcohol you must get from your doctor drugs for the transition period between drinking alcohol and abstinence. Abrupt stop of drinking alcohol can be very dangerous for your health and even life.

***

Night

Before sleep

- Take a shower (warm water) 1 min.
- Small physical excercise 3 min.

In Bed

- Repeat STOP (20 times)
- Say slowly untill you fall asleep: sun, flower, seven, path, tee, run, yellow, apple, fish, rain, pen, water, smile, talk, life, sky.

If you cannot fall asleep

- Say slowly untill you fall asleep: sun, flower, seven, path, tee, run, yellow, apple, fish, rain, pen, water, smile, talk, life, sky.

If above does not help

- Stand up and go to the toilet (when possible with as little light as possible)
- Say slowly untill you fall asleep: sun, flower, seven, path, tee, run, yellow, apple, fish, rain, pen, water, smile, talk, life, sky.

If above does not help

- Say STOP untill you fall asleep

If above does not help

- Go to the kitchen and have a very small snack.
- Back to the bed say slowly untill you fall asleep: sun, flower, seven, path, tee, run, yellow, apple, fish, rain, pen, water, smile, talk, life, sky.

If above does not help

- Say slowly untill morning: sun, flower, seven, path, tee, run, yellow, apple, fish, rain, pen, water, smile, talk, life, sky.

***

Day 2

Morning

* Repeat STOP (10 times every 30 min)

* Say slowly every hour: sun, flower, seven, path, tee, run, yellow, apple, fish, rain, pen, water, smile, talk, life, sky.

* Small physical excercise (10 min)

* Small breakfast.

* Nice talk (no complaints) 20 min. When nobody to talk with, phone or internet conversation oral or written.

* Walk 15 min.

* Every time the desire to drink alcohol comes back to you, imagine that you want to continue without alcohol only a little bit more. Never think that you will never ever drink alcohol again. Of course this would be great but for some people it is impossible to stand the idea, especially at the beginning of the therapy. But instead of breaking the abstinence right away, ALWAYS give yourself some time, even very short and say to yourself:

I will wait still one hour.

I will wait still 2 hours.

I will wait still 3 hours.

Etc.

I will wait still one day.

I will wait still 2 days.

I will wait still 3 days.

Etc.

Afer one hour or 2 hours or one day or 2 days passed by, ask yourself:

Do I feel the desire to drink alcohol?

No

In such a case you can continue with abstinence untill next time you feel the desire to drink alcohol.

Yes

In such a case you can make one more effort and one more time put untill later drinking alcohol again. Are you ready to make such an effort?

Yes

In this case you continue the abstinence.

No

In this case you are close to loose this time the battle with alcohol. This means you are not yet determined enough to continue the abstinence.

Try again later and never think when giving up drinking alcohol that it is for always. Always think it is for as long as possible.

Attention! Every time you give up alcohol you must get from your doctor drugs for the transition period between drinking alcohol and abstinence. Abrupt stop of drinking alcohol can be very dangerous for your health and even life.

***

Afternoon

* Repeat STOP (10 times every 30 min.)

* Say slowly every hour: sun, flower, seven, path, tee, run, yellow, apple, fish, rain, pen, water, smile, talk, life, sky.

* Dinner and half an hour break (you can sleep).

* Nice talk (no complaints) 30 min. When nobody to talk with, phone or internet conversation oral or written.

* Walk 15 min.

* Every time the desire to drink alcohol comes back to you, imagine that you want to continue without alcohol only a little bit more. Never think that you will never ever drink alcohol again. Of course this would be great but for some people it is impossible to stand the idea, especially at the beginning of the therapy. But instead of breaking the abstinence right away, ALWAYS give yourself some time, even very short and say to yourself:

I will wait still one hour.

I will wait still 2 hours.

I will wait still 3 hours.

Etc.

I will wait still one day.

I will wait still 2 days.

I will wait still 3 days.

Etc.

Afer one hour or 2 hours or one day or 2 days passed by, ask yourself:

Do I feel the desire to drink alcohol?

No

In such a case you can continue with abstinence untill next time you feel the desire to drink alcohol.

Yes

In such a case you can make one more effort and one more time put untill later drinking alcohol again. Are you ready to make such an effort?

Yes

In this case you continue the abstinence.

No

In this case you are close to loose this time the battle with alcohol. This means you are not yet determined enough to continue the abstinence.

Try again later and never think when giving up drinking alcohol that it is for always. Always think it is for as long as possible.

Attention! Every time you give up alcohol you must get from your doctor drugs for the transition period between drinking alcohol and abstinence. Abrupt stop of drinking alcohol can be very dangerous for your health and even life.

***

Evening

- Repeat STOP (10 times every 30 min.)
- Say slowly every hour: sun, flower, seven, path, tee, run, yellow, apple, fish, rain, pen, water, smile, talk, life, sky.
- Small supper.
- Nice talk (no complaints) 20 min. When nobody to talk with, phone or internet conversation oral or written.
- Walk 15 min.
- Every time the desire to drink alcohol comes back to you, imagine that you want to continue without alcohol only a little bit more. Never think that you will never ever drink alcohol again. Of course this would be great but for some people it is impossible to stand the idea, especially at the beginning of the therapy. But instead of breaking the abstinence right away,

ALWAYS give yourself some time, even very short and say to yourself:

I will wait still one hour.
I will wait still 2 hours.
I will wait still 3 hours.
Etc.
I will wait still one day.
I will wait still 2 days.
I will wait still 3 days.
Etc.

Afer one hour or 2 hours or one day or 2 days passed by, ask yourself:

Do I feel the desire to drink alcohol?

No

In such a case you can continue with abstinence untill next time you feel the desire to drink alcohol.

Yes

In such a case you can make one more effort and one more time put untill later drinking alcohol again. Are you ready to make such an effort?

Yes

In this case you continue the abstinence.

No

In this case you are close to loose this time the battle with alcohol. This means you are not yet determined enough to continue the abstinence. Try again later and never think when giving up drinking alcohol that it is for always. Always think it is for as long as possible.

Attention! Every time you give up alcohol you must get from your doctor drugs for the transition period between drinking alcohol and abstinence. Abrupt stop of drinking alcohol can be very dangerous for your health and even life.

***

Night

Before sleep

- Take a shower (warm water) 1 min.
- Small physical excercise 3 min.

In Bed

- Repeat STOP (20 times)
- Say slowly untill you fall asleep: sun, flower, seven, path, tee, run, yellow, apple, fish, rain, pen, water, smile, talk, life, sky.

If you cannot fall asleep

- Say slowly untill you fall asleep: sun, flower, seven, path, tee, run, yellow, apple, fish, rain, pen, water, smile, talk, life, sky.

If above does not help

- Stand up and go to the toilet (when possible with as little light as possible)
- Say slowly untill you fall asleep: sun, flower, seven, path, tee, run, yellow, apple, fish, rain, pen, water, smile, talk, life, sky.

If above does not help

- Say STOP untill you fall asleep

If above does not help

- Go to the kitchen and have a very small snack.
- Back to the bed say slowly untill you fall asleep: sun, flower, seven, path, tee, run, yellow, apple, fish, rain, pen, water, smile, talk, life, sky.

If above does not help

- Say slowly untill morning: sun, flower, seven, path, tee, run, yellow, apple, fish, rain, pen, water, smile, talk, life, sky.

***

Day 3

Morning

* Repeat STOP (10 times every 30 min)

* Say slowly every hour: sun, flower, seven, path, tee, run, yellow, apple, fish, rain, pen, water, smile, talk, life, sky.

* Small physical excercise (10 min)

* Small breakfast.

* Nice talk (no complaints) 20 min. When nobody to talk with, phone or internet conversation oral or written.

* Walk 15 min.

* Every time the desire to drink alcohol comes back to you, imagine that you want to continue without alcohol only a little bit more. Never think that you will never ever drink alcohol again. Of course this would be great but for some people it is impossible to stand the idea, especially at the beginning of the therapy. But instead of breaking the abstinence right away, ALWAYS give yourself some time, even very short and say to yourself:

I will wait still one hour.

I will wait still 2 hours.

I will wait still 3 hours.

Etc.

I will wait still one day.

I will wait still 2 days.

I will wait still 3 days.

Etc.

Afer one hour or 2 hours or one day or 2 days passed by, ask yourself:

Do I feel the desire to drink alcohol?

No

In such a case you can continue with abstinence untill next time you feel the desire to drink alcohol.

Yes

In such a case you can make one more effort and one more time put untill later drinking alcohol again. Are you ready to make such an effort?

Yes

In this case you continue the abstinence.

No

In this case you are close to loose this time the battle with alcohol. This means you are not yet determined enough to continue the abstinence.

Try again later and never think when giving up drinking alcohol that it is for always. Always think it is for as long as possible.

Attention! Every time you give up alcohol you must get from your doctor drugs for the transition period between drinking alcohol and abstinence. Abrupt stop of drinking alcohol can be very dangerous for your health and even life.

***

Afternoon

* Repeat STOP (10 times every 30 min.)

* Say slowly every hour: sun, flower, seven, path, tee, run, yellow, apple, fish, rain, pen, water, smile, talk, life, sky.

* Dinner and half an hour break (you can sleep).

* Nice talk (no complaints) 30 min. When nobody to talk with, phone or internet conversation oral or written.

* Walk 15 min.

* Every time the desire to drink alcohol comes back to you, imagine that you want to continue without alcohol only a little bit more. Never think that you will never

ever drink alcohol again. Of course this would be great but for some people it is impossible to stand the idea, especially at the beginning of the therapy. But instead of breaking the abstinence right away, ALWAYS give yourself some time, even very short and say to yourself:

I will wait still one hour.

I will wait still 2 hours.

I will wait still 3 hours.

Etc.

I will wait still one day.

I will wait still 2 days.

I will wait still 3 days.

Etc.

Afer one hour or 2 hours or one day or 2 days passed by, ask yourself:

Do I feel the desire to drink alcohol?

No

In such a case you can continue with abstinence untill next time you feel the desire to drink alcohol.

Yes

In such a case you can make one more effort and one more time put untill later drinking alcohol again. Are you ready to make such an effort?

Yes

In this case you continue the abstinence.

No

In this case you are close to loose this time the battle with alcohol. This means you are not yet determined enough to continue the abstinence.

Try again later and never think when giving up drinking alcohol that it is for always. Always think it is for as long as possible.

Attention! Every time you give up alcohol you must get from your doctor drugs for the transition period between drinking alcohol and abstinence. Abrupt stop of drinking alcohol can be very dangerous for your health and even life.

***

Evening

- Repeat STOP (10 times every 30 min.)
- Say slowly every hour: sun, flower, seven, path, tee, run, yellow, apple, fish, rain, pen, water, smile, talk, life, sky.

- Small supper.
- Nice talk (no complaints) 20 min. When nobody to talk with, phone or internet conversation oral or written.
- Walk 15 min.
- Every time the desire to drink alcohol comes back to you, imagine that you want to continue without alcohol only a little bit more. Never think that you will never ever drink alcohol again. Of course this would be great but for some people it is impossible to stand the idea, especially at the beginning of the therapy. But instead of breaking the abstinence right away, ALWAYS give yourself some time, even very short and say to yourself:

  I will wait still one hour.

  I will wait still 2 hours.

  I will wait still 3 hours.

  Etc.

  I will wait still one day.

  I will wait still 2 days.

  I will wait still 3 days.

  Etc.

  Afer one hour or 2 hours or one day or 2 days passed by, ask yourself:

  Do I feel the desire to drink alcohol?

No

In such a case you can continue with abstinence untill next time you feel the desire to drink alcohol.

Yes

In such a case you can make one more effort and one more time put untill later drinking alcohol again. Are you ready to make such an effort?

Yes

In this case you continue the abstinence.

No

In this case you are close to loose this time the battle with alcohol. This means you are not yet determined enough to continue the abstinence. Try again later and never think when giving up drinking alcohol that it is for always. Always think it is for as long as possible.

Attention! Every time you give up alcohol you must get from your doctor drugs for the transition period between drinking alcohol and abstinence. Abrupt stop of drinking alcohol can be very dangerous for your health and even life.

***

Night

Before sleep

- Take a shower (warm water) 1 min.
- Small physical excercise 3 min.

In Bed

- Repeat STOP (20 times)
- Say slowly untill you fall asleep: sun, flower, seven, path, tee, run, yellow, apple, fish, rain, pen, water, smile, talk, life, sky.

If you cannot fall asleep

- Say slowly untill you fall asleep: sun, flower, seven, path, tee, run, yellow, apple, fish, rain, pen, water, smile, talk, life, sky.

If above does not help

- Stand up and go to the toilet (when possible with as little light as possible)
- Say slowly untill you fall asleep: sun, flower, seven, path, tee, run, yellow, apple, fish, rain, pen, water, smile, talk, life, sky.

If above does not help

- Say STOP untill you fall asleep

If above does not help

- Go to the kitchen and have a very small snack.

- Back to the bed say slowly untill you fall asleep: sun, flower, seven, path, tee, run, yellow, apple, fish, rain, pen, water, smile, talk, life, sky.

If above does not help

- Say slowly untill morning: sun, flower, seven, path, tee, run, yellow, apple, fish, rain, pen, water, smile, talk, life, sky.

***

Day 4

Morning

* Repeat STOP (10 times every 30 min)

* Say slowly every hour: sun, flower, seven, path, tee, run, yellow, apple, fish, rain, pen, water, smile, talk, life, sky.

* Small physical excercise (10 min)

* Small breakfast.

* Nice talk (no complaints) 20 min. When nobody to talk with, phone or internet conversation oral or written.

* Walk 15 min.

* Every time the desire to drink alcohol comes back to you, imagine that you want to continue without alcohol

only a little bit more. Never think that you will never ever drink alcohol again. Of course this would be great but for some people it is impossible to stand the idea, especially at the beginning of the therapy. But instead of breaking the abstinence right away, ALWAYS give yourself some time, even very short and say to yourself:

I will wait still one hour.

I will wait still 2 hours.

I will wait still 3 hours.

Etc.

I will wait still one day.

I will wait still 2 days.

I will wait still 3 days.

Etc.

Afer one hour or 2 hours or one day or 2 days passed by, ask yourself:

Do I feel the desire to drink alcohol?

No

In such a case you can continue with abstinence untill next time you feel the desire to drink alcohol.

Yes

In such a case you can make one more effort and one more time put untill later drinking alcohol again. Are you ready to make such an effort?

Yes

In this case you continue the abstinence.

No

In this case you are close to loose this time the battle with alcohol. This means you are not yet determined enough to continue the abstinence.

Try again later and never think when giving up drinking alcohol that it is for always. Always think it is for as long as possible.

Attention! Every time you give up alcohol you must get from your doctor drugs for the transition period between drinking alcohol and abstinence. Abrupt stop of drinking alcohol can be very dangerous for your health and even life.

***

Afternoon

* Repeat STOP (10 times every 30 min.)

* Say slowly every hour: sun, flower, seven, path, tee, run, yellow, apple, fish, rain, pen, water, smile, talk, life, sky.

* Dinner and half an hour break (you can sleep).

* Nice talk (no complaints) 30 min. When nobody to talk with, phone or internet conversation oral or written.

* Walk 15 min.

* Every time the desire to drink alcohol comes back to you, imagine that you want to continue without alcohol only a little bit more. Never think that you will never ever drink alcohol again. Of course this would be great but for some people it is impossible to stand the idea, especially at the beginning of the therapy. But instead of breaking the abstinence right away, ALWAYS give yourself some time, even very short and say to yourself:

I will wait still one hour.

I will wait still 2 hours.

I will wait still 3 hours.

Etc.

I will wait still one day.

I will wait still 2 days.

I will wait still 3 days.

Etc.

Afer one hour or 2 hours or one day or 2 days passed by, ask yourself:

Do I feel the desire to drink alcohol?

No

In such a case you can continue with abstinence untill next time you feel the desire to drink alcohol.

Yes

In such a case you can make one more effort and one more time put untill later drinking alcohol again. Are you ready to make such an effort?

Yes

In this case you continue the abstinence.

No

In this case you are close to loose this time the battle with alcohol. This means you are not yet determined enough to continue the abstinence.

Try again later and never think when giving up drinking alcohol that it is for always. Always think it is for as long as possible.

Attention! Every time you give up alcohol you must get from your doctor drugs for the transition period between drinking alcohol and abstinence. Abrupt stop of drinking alcohol can be very dangerous for your health and even life.

***

Evening

- Repeat STOP (10 times every 30 min.)
- Say slowly every hour: sun, flower, seven, path, tee, run, yellow, apple, fish, rain, pen, water, smile, talk, life, sky.
- Small supper.
- Nice talk (no complaints) 20 min. When nobody to talk with, phone or internet conversation oral or written.
- Walk 15 min.
- Every time the desire to drink alcohol comes back to you, imagine that you want to continue without alcohol only a little bit more. Never think that you will never ever drink alcohol again. Of course this would be great but for some people it is impossible to stand the idea, especially at the beginning of the therapy. But instead of breaking the abstinence right away,

ALWAYS give yourself some time, even very short and say to yourself:

I will wait still one hour.

I will wait still 2 hours.

I will wait still 3 hours.

Etc.

I will wait still one day.

I will wait still 2 days.

I will wait still 3 days.

Etc.

Afer one hour or 2 hours or one day or 2 days passed by, ask yourself:

Do I feel the desire to drink alcohol?

No

In such a case you can continue with abstinence untill next time you feel the desire to drink alcohol.

Yes

In such a case you can make one more effort and one more time put untill later drinking alcohol again. Are you ready to make such an effort?

Yes

In this case you continue the abstinence.

No

In this case you are close to loose this time the battle with alcohol. This means you are not yet determined enough to continue the abstinence. Try again later and never think when giving up drinking alcohol that it is for always. Always think it is for as long as possible.

Attention! Every time you give up alcohol you must get from your doctor drugs for the transition period between drinking alcohol and abstinence. Abrupt stop of drinking alcohol can be very dangerous for your health and even life.

***

Night

Before sleep

- Take a shower (warm water) 1 min.
- Small physical excercise 3 min.

In Bed

- Repeat STOP (20 times)
- Say slowly untill you fall asleep: sun, flower, seven, path, tee, run, yellow, apple, fish, rain, pen, water, smile, talk, life, sky.

If you cannot fall asleep

- Say slowly untill you fall asleep: sun, flower, seven, path, tee, run, yellow, apple, fish, rain, pen, water, smile, talk, life, sky.

If above does not help

- Stand up and go to the toilet (when possible with as little light as possible)
- Say slowly untill you fall asleep: sun, flower, seven, path, tee, run, yellow, apple, fish, rain, pen, water, smile, talk, life, sky.

If above does not help

- Say STOP untill you fall asleep

If above does not help

- Go to the kitchen and have a very small snack.
- Back to the bed say slowly untill you fall asleep: sun, flower, seven, path, tee, run, yellow, apple, fish, rain, pen, water, smile, talk, life, sky.

If above does not help

- Say slowly untill morning: sun, flower, seven, path, tee, run, yellow, apple, fish, rain, pen, water, smile, talk, life, sky.

***

Day 5

Morning

* Repeat STOP (10 times every 30 min)

* Say slowly every hour: sun, flower, seven, path, tee, run, yellow, apple, fish, rain, pen, water, smile, talk, life, sky.

* Small physical excercise (10 min)

* Small breakfast.

* Nice talk (no complaints) 20 min. When nobody to talk with, phone or internet conversation oral or written.

* Walk 15 min.

* Every time the desire to drink alcohol comes back to you, imagine that you want to continue without alcohol only a little bit more. Never think that you will never ever drink alcohol again. Of course this would be great but for some people it is impossible to stand the idea, especially at the beginning of the therapy. But instead of breaking the abstinence right away, ALWAYS give yourself some time, even very short and say to yourself:

I will wait still one hour.

I will wait still 2 hours.

I will wait still 3 hours.

Etc.

I will wait still one day.

I will wait still 2 days.

I will wait still 3 days.

Etc.

Afer one hour or 2 hours or one day or 2 days passed by, ask yourself:

Do I feel the desire to drink alcohol?

No

In such a case you can continue with abstinence untill next time you feel the desire to drink alcohol.

Yes

In such a case you can make one more effort and one more time put untill later drinking alcohol again. Are you ready to make such an effort?

Yes

In this case you continue the abstinence.

No

In this case you are close to loose this time the battle with alcohol. This means you are not yet determined enough to continue the abstinence.

Try again later and never think when giving up drinking alcohol that it is for always. Always think it is for as long as possible.

Attention! Every time you give up alcohol you must get from your doctor drugs for the transition period between drinking alcohol and abstinence. Abrupt stop of drinking alcohol can be very dangerous for your health and even life.

***

Afternoon

* Repeat STOP (10 times every 30 min.)

* Say slowly every hour: sun, flower, seven, path, tee, run, yellow, apple, fish, rain, pen, water, smile, talk, life, sky.

* Dinner and half an hour break (you can sleep).

* Nice talk (no complaints) 30 min. When nobody to talk with, phone or internet conversation oral or written.

* Walk 15 min.

* Every time the desire to drink alcohol comes back to you, imagine that you want to continue without alcohol only a little bit more. Never think that you will never

ever drink alcohol again. Of course this would be great but for some people it is impossible to stand the idea, especially at the beginning of the therapy. But instead of breaking the abstinence right away, ALWAYS give yourself some time, even very short and say to yourself:

I will wait still one hour.

I will wait still 2 hours.

I will wait still 3 hours.

Etc.

I will wait still one day.

I will wait still 2 days.

I will wait still 3 days.

Etc.

Afer one hour or 2 hours or one day or 2 days passed by, ask yourself:

Do I feel the desire to drink alcohol?

No

In such a case you can continue with abstinence untill next time you feel the desire to drink alcohol.

Yes

In such a case you can make one more effort and one more time put untill later drinking alcohol again. Are you ready to make such an effort?

Yes

In this case you continue the abstinence.

No

In this case you are close to loose this time the battle with alcohol. This means you are not yet determined enough to continue the abstinence.

Try again later and never think when giving up drinking alcohol that it is for always. Always think it is for as long as possible.

Attention! Every time you give up alcohol you must get from your doctor drugs for the transition period between drinking alcohol and abstinence. Abrupt stop of drinking alcohol can be very dangerous for your health and even life.

***

Evening

- Repeat STOP (10 times every 30 min.)
- Say slowly every hour: sun, flower, seven, path, tee, run, yellow, apple, fish, rain, pen, water, smile, talk, life, sky.

- Small supper.
- Nice talk (no complaints) 20 min. When nobody to talk with, phone or internet conversation oral or written.
- Walk 15 min.
- Every time the desire to drink alcohol comes back to you, imagine that you want to continue without alcohol only a little bit more. Never think that you will never ever drink alcohol again. Of course this would be great but for some people it is impossible to stand the idea, especially at the beginning of the therapy. But instead of breaking the abstinence right away, ALWAYS give yourself some time, even very short and say to yourself:

  I will wait still one hour.

  I will wait still 2 hours.

  I will wait still 3 hours.

  Etc.

  I will wait still one day.

  I will wait still 2 days.

  I will wait still 3 days.

  Etc.

  Afer one hour or 2 hours or one day or 2 days passed by, ask yourself:

  Do I feel the desire to drink alcohol?

No

In such a case you can continue with abstinence untill next time you feel the desire to drink alcohol.

Yes

In such a case you can make one more effort and one more time put untill later drinking alcohol again. Are you ready to make such an effort?

Yes

In this case you continue the abstinence.

No

In this case you are close to loose this time the battle with alcohol. This means you are not yet determined enough to continue the abstinence. Try again later and never think when giving up drinking alcohol that it is for always. Always think it is for as long as possible.

Attention! Every time you give up alcohol you must get from your doctor drugs for the transition period between drinking alcohol and abstinence. Abrupt stop of drinking alcohol can be very dangerous for your health and even life.

***

Night

Before sleep

- Take a shower (warm water) 1 min.
- Small physical excercise 3 min.

In Bed

- Repeat STOP (20 times)
- Say slowly untill you fall asleep: sun, flower, seven, path, tee, run, yellow, apple, fish, rain, pen, water, smile, talk, life, sky.

If you cannot fall asleep

- Say slowly untill you fall asleep: sun, flower, seven, path, tee, run, yellow, apple, fish, rain, pen, water, smile, talk, life, sky.

If above does not help

- Stand up and go to the toilet (when possible with as little light as possible)
- Say slowly untill you fall asleep: sun, flower, seven, path, tee, run, yellow, apple, fish, rain, pen, water, smile, talk, life, sky.

If above does not help

- Say STOP untill you fall asleep

If above does not help

- Go to the kitchen and have a very small snack.

- Back to the bed say slowly untill you fall asleep: sun, flower, seven, path, tee, run, yellow, apple, fish, rain, pen, water, smile, talk, life, sky.

If above does not help

- Say slowly untill morning: sun, flower, seven, path, tee, run, yellow, apple, fish, rain, pen, water, smile, talk, life, sky.

***

Day 6

Morning

* Repeat STOP (10 times every 30 min)

* Say slowly every hour: sun, flower, seven, path, tee, run, yellow, apple, fish, rain, pen, water, smile, talk, life, sky.

* Small physical excercise (10 min)

* Small breakfast.

* Nice talk (no complaints) 20 min. When nobody to talk with, phone or internet conversation oral or written.

* Walk 15 min.

* Every time the desire to drink alcohol comes back to you, imagine that you want to continue without alcohol

only a little bit more. Never think that you will never ever drink alcohol again. Of course this would be great but for some people it is impossible to stand the idea, especially at the beginning of the therapy. But instead of breaking the abstinence right away, ALWAYS give yourself some time, even very short and say to yourself:

I will wait still one hour.

I will wait still 2 hours.

I will wait still 3 hours.

Etc.

I will wait still one day.

I will wait still 2 days.

I will wait still 3 days.

Etc.

Afer one hour or 2 hours or one day or 2 days passed by, ask yourself:

Do I feel the desire to drink alcohol?

No

In such a case you can continue with abstinence untill next time you feel the desire to drink alcohol.

Yes

In such a case you can make one more effort and one more time put untill later drinking alcohol again. Are you ready to make such an effort?

Yes

In this case you continue the abstinence.

No

In this case you are close to loose this time the battle with alcohol. This means you are not yet determined enough to continue the abstinence.

Try again later and never think when giving up drinking alcohol that it is for always. Always think it is for as long as possible.

Attention! Every time you give up alcohol you must get from your doctor drugs for the transition period between drinking alcohol and abstinence. Abrupt stop of drinking alcohol can be very dangerous for your health and even life.

***

Afternoon

* Repeat STOP (10 times every 30 min.)

* Say slowly every hour: sun, flower, seven, path, tee, run, yellow, apple, fish, rain, pen, water, smile, talk, life, sky.

* Dinner and half an hour break (you can sleep).

* Nice talk (no complaints) 30 min. When nobody to talk with, phone or internet conversation oral or written.

* Walk 15 min.

* Every time the desire to drink alcohol comes back to you, imagine that you want to continue without alcohol only a little bit more. Never think that you will never ever drink alcohol again. Of course this would be great but for some people it is impossible to stand the idea, especially at the beginning of the therapy. But instead of breaking the abstinence right away, ALWAYS give yourself some time, even very short and say to yourself:

I will wait still one hour.

I will wait still 2 hours.

I will wait still 3 hours.

Etc.

I will wait still one day.

I will wait still 2 days.

I will wait still 3 days.

Etc.

Afer one hour or 2 hours or one day or 2 days passed by, ask yourself:

Do I feel the desire to drink alcohol?

No

In such a case you can continue with abstinence untill next time you feel the desire to drink alcohol.

Yes

In such a case you can make one more effort and one more time put untill later drinking alcohol again. Are you ready to make such an effort?

Yes

In this case you continue the abstinence.

No

In this case you are close to loose this time the battle with alcohol. This means you are not yet determined enough to continue the abstinence.

Try again later and never think when giving up drinking alcohol that it is for always. Always think it is for as long as possible.

Attention! Every time you give up alcohol you must get from your doctor drugs for the transition period between drinking alcohol and abstinence. Abrupt stop of drinking alcohol can be very dangerous for your health and even life.

***

Evening

- Repeat STOP (10 times every 30 min.)
- Say slowly every hour: sun, flower, seven, path, tee, run, yellow, apple, fish, rain, pen, water, smile, talk, life, sky.
- Small supper.
- Nice talk (no complaints) 20 min. When nobody to talk with, phone or internet conversation oral or written.
- Walk 15 min.
- Every time the desire to drink alcohol comes back to you, imagine that you want to continue without alcohol only a little bit more. Never think that you will never ever drink alcohol again. Of course this would be great but for some people it is impossible to stand the idea, especially at the beginning of the therapy. But instead of breaking the abstinence right away,

ALWAYS give yourself some time, even very short and say to yourself:

I will wait still one hour.
I will wait still 2 hours.
I will wait still 3 hours.
Etc.
I will wait still one day.
I will wait still 2 days.
I will wait still 3 days.
Etc.

Afer one hour or 2 hours or one day or 2 days passed by, ask yourself:

Do I feel the desire to drink alcohol?

No

In such a case you can continue with abstinence untill next time you feel the desire to drink alcohol.

Yes

In such a case you can make one more effort and one more time put untill later drinking alcohol again. Are you ready to make such an effort?

Yes

In this case you continue the abstinence.

No

In this case you are close to loose this time the battle with alcohol. This means you are not yet determined enough to continue the abstinence. Try again later and never think when giving up drinking alcohol that it is for always. Always think it is for as long as possible.

Attention! Every time you give up alcohol you must get from your doctor drugs for the transition period between drinking alcohol and abstinence. Abrupt stop of drinking alcohol can be very dangerous for your health and even life.

***

Night

Before sleep

- Take a shower (warm water) 1 min.
- Small physical excercise 3 min.

In Bed

- Repeat STOP (20 times)
- Say slowly untill you fall asleep: sun, flower, seven, path, tee, run, yellow, apple, fish, rain, pen, water, smile, talk, life, sky.

If you cannot fall asleep

- Say slowly untill you fall asleep: sun, flower, seven, path, tee, run, yellow, apple, fish, rain, pen, water, smile, talk, life, sky.

If above does not help

- Stand up and go to the toilet (when possible with as little light as possible)
- Say slowly untill you fall asleep: sun, flower, seven, path, tee, run, yellow, apple, fish, rain, pen, water, smile, talk, life, sky.

If above does not help

- Say STOP untill you fall asleep

If above does not help

- Go to the kitchen and have a very small snack.
- Back to the bed say slowly untill you fall asleep: sun, flower, seven, path, tee, run, yellow, apple, fish, rain, pen, water, smile, talk, life, sky.

If above does not help

- Say slowly untill morning: sun, flower, seven, path, tee, run, yellow, apple, fish, rain, pen, water, smile, talk, life, sky.

***

Day 7

Morning

* Repeat STOP (10 times every 30 min)

* Say slowly every hour: sun, flower, seven, path, tee, run, yellow, apple, fish, rain, pen, water, smile, talk, life, sky.

* Small physical excercise (10 min)

* Small breakfast.

* Nice talk (no complaints) 20 min. When nobody to talk with, phone or internet conversation oral or written.

* Walk 15 min.

* Every time the desire to drink alcohol comes back to you, imagine that you want to continue without alcohol only a little bit more. Never think that you will never ever drink alcohol again. Of course this would be great but for some people it is impossible to stand the idea, especially at the beginning of the therapy. But instead of breaking the abstinence right away, ALWAYS give yourself some time, even very short and say to yourself:

I will wait still one hour.

I will wait still 2 hours.

I will wait still 3 hours.

Etc.

I will wait still one day.

I will wait still 2 days.

I will wait still 3 days.

Etc.

Afer one hour or 2 hours or one day or 2 days passed by, ask yourself:

Do I feel the desire to drink alcohol?

No

In such a case you can continue with abstinence untill next time you feel the desire to drink alcohol.

Yes

In such a case you can make one more effort and one more time put untill later drinking alcohol again. Are you ready to make such an effort?

Yes

In this case you continue the abstinence.

No

In this case you are close to loose this time the battle with alcohol. This means you are not yet determined enough to continue the abstinence.

Try again later and never think when giving up drinking alcohol that it is for always. Always think it is for as long as possible.

Attention! Every time you give up alcohol you must get from your doctor drugs for the transition period between drinking alcohol and abstinence. Abrupt stop of drinking alcohol can be very dangerous for your health and even life.

***

Afternoon

* Repeat STOP (10 times every 30 min.)

* Say slowly every hour: sun, flower, seven, path, tee, run, yellow, apple, fish, rain, pen, water, smile, talk, life, sky.

* Dinner and half an hour break (you can sleep).

* Nice talk (no complaints) 30 min. When nobody to talk with, phone or internet conversation oral or written.

* Walk 15 min.

* Every time the desire to drink alcohol comes back to you, imagine that you want to continue without alcohol only a little bit more. Never think that you will never

ever drink alcohol again. Of course this would be great but for some people it is impossible to stand the idea, especially at the beginning of the therapy. But instead of breaking the abstinence right away, ALWAYS give yourself some time, even very short and say to yourself:

I will wait still one hour.

I will wait still 2 hours.

I will wait still 3 hours.

Etc.

I will wait still one day.

I will wait still 2 days.

I will wait still 3 days.

Etc.

Afer one hour or 2 hours or one day or 2 days passed by, ask yourself:

Do I feel the desire to drink alcohol?

No

In such a case you can continue with abstinence untill next time you feel the desire to drink alcohol.

Yes

In such a case you can make one more effort and one more time put untill later drinking alcohol again. Are you ready to make such an effort?

Yes

In this case you continue the abstinence.

No

In this case you are close to loose this time the battle with alcohol. This means you are not yet determined enough to continue the abstinence.

Try again later and never think when giving up drinking alcohol that it is for always. Always think it is for as long as possible.

Attention! Every time you give up alcohol you must get from your doctor drugs for the transition period between drinking alcohol and abstinence. Abrupt stop of drinking alcohol can be very dangerous for your health and even life.

***

Evening

- Repeat STOP (10 times every 30 min.)
- Say slowly every hour: sun, flower, seven, path, tee, run, yellow, apple, fish, rain, pen, water, smile, talk, life, sky.

- Small supper.
- Nice talk (no complaints) 20 min. When nobody to talk with, phone or internet conversation oral or written.
- Walk 15 min.
- Every time the desire to drink alcohol comes back to you, imagine that you want to continue without alcohol only a little bit more. Never think that you will never ever drink alcohol again. Of course this would be great but for some people it is impossible to stand the idea, especially at the beginning of the therapy. But instead of breaking the abstinence right away, ALWAYS give yourself some time, even very short and say to yourself:

  I will wait still one hour.

  I will wait still 2 hours.

  I will wait still 3 hours.

  Etc.

  I will wait still one day.

  I will wait still 2 days.

  I will wait still 3 days.

  Etc.

  Afer one hour or 2 hours or one day or 2 days passed by, ask yourself:

  Do I feel the desire to drink alcohol?

No

In such a case you can continue with abstinence untill next time you feel the desire to drink alcohol.

Yes

In such a case you can make one more effort and one more time put untill later drinking alcohol again. Are you ready to make such an effort?

Yes

In this case you continue the abstinence.

No

In this case you are close to loose this time the battle with alcohol. This means you are not yet determined enough to continue the abstinence. Try again later and never think when giving up drinking alcohol that it is for always. Always think it is for as long as possible.

Attention! Every time you give up alcohol you must get from your doctor drugs for the transition period between drinking alcohol and abstinence. Abrupt stop of drinking alcohol can be very dangerous for your health and even life.

***

Night

Before sleep

- Take a shower (warm water) 1 min.
- Small physical excercise 3 min.

In Bed

- Repeat STOP (20 times)
- Say slowly untill you fall asleep: sun, flower, seven, path, tee, run, yellow, apple, fish, rain, pen, water, smile, talk, life, sky.

If you cannot fall asleep

- Say slowly untill you fall asleep: sun, flower, seven, path, tee, run, yellow, apple, fish, rain, pen, water, smile, talk, life, sky.

If above does not help

- Stand up and go to the toilet (when possible with as little light as possible)
- Say slowly untill you fall asleep: sun, flower, seven, path, tee, run, yellow, apple, fish, rain, pen, water, smile, talk, life, sky.

If above does not help

- Say STOP untill you fall asleep

If above does not help

- Go to the kitchen and have a very small snack.

- Back to the bed say slowly untill you fall asleep: sun, flower, seven, path, tee, run, yellow, apple, fish, rain, pen, water, smile, talk, life, sky.

If above does not help

- Say slowly untill morning: sun, flower, seven, path, tee, run, yellow, apple, fish, rain, pen, water, smile, talk, life, sky.

***

Week Two

***

Day 1

Morning

* Repeat STOP (10 times every hour)

* Say slowly every 2 hours: sun, flower, seven, path, tee, run, yellow, apple, fish, rain, pen, water, smile, talk, life, sky.

* Small physical excercise (15 min)

* Small breakfast.

* Nice talk (no complaints) 25 min. When nobody to talk with, phone or internet conversation oral or written.

* Walk 20 min.

* Every time the desire to drink alcohol comes back to you, imagine that you want to continue without alcohol only a little bit more. Never think that you will never ever drink alcohol again. Of course this would be great but for some people it is impossible to stand the idea, especially at the beginning of the therapy. But instead of breaking the abstinence right away, ALWAYS give yourself some time, even very short and say to yourself:

I will wait still one hour.

I will wait still 2 hours.

I will wait still 3 hours.

Etc.

I will wait still one day.

I will wait still 2 days.

I will wait still 3 days.

Etc.

Afer one hour or 2 hours or one day or 2 days passed by, ask yourself:

Do I feel the desire to drink alcohol?

No

In such a case you can continue with abstinence untill next time you feel the desire to drink alcohol.

Yes

In such a case you can make one more effort and one more time put untill later drinking alcohol again. Are you ready to make such an effort?

Yes

In this case you continue the abstinence.

No

In this case you are close to loose this time the battle with alcohol. This means you are not yet determined enough to continue the abstinence.

Try again later and never think when giving up drinking alcohol that it is for always. Always think it is for as long as possible.

Attention! Every time you give up alcohol you must get from your doctor drugs for the transition period between drinking alcohol and abstinence. Abrupt stop of drinking alcohol can be very dangerous for your health and even life.

***

Afternoon

* Repeat STOP (10 times every hour.)

* Say slowly every 2 hours: sun, flower, seven, path, tee, run, yellow, apple, fish, rain, pen, water, smile, talk, life, sky.

* Dinner and half an hour break (you can sleep).

* Nice talk (no complaints) 30 min. When nobody to talk with, phone or internet conversation oral or written.

* Walk 20 min.

* Every time the desire to drink alcohol comes back to you, imagine that you want to continue without alcohol only a little bit more. Never think that you will never ever drink alcohol again. Of course this would be great but for some people it is impossible to stand the idea, especially at the beginning of the therapy. But instead of breaking the abstinence right away, ALWAYS give yourself some time, even very short and say to yourself:

I will wait still one hour.

I will wait still 2 hours.

I will wait still 3 hours.

Etc.

I will wait still one day.

I will wait still 2 days.

I will wait still 3 days.

Etc.

Afer one hour or 2 hours or one day or 2 days passed by, ask yourself:

Do I feel the desire to drink alcohol?

No

In such a case you can continue with abstinence untill next time you feel the desire to drink alcohol.

Yes

In such a case you can make one more effort and one more time put untill later drinking alcohol again. Are you ready to make such an effort?

Yes

In this case you continue the abstinence.

No

In this case you are close to loose this time the battle with alcohol. This means you are not yet determined enough to continue the abstinence.

Try again later and never think when giving up drinking alcohol that it is for always. Always think it is for as long as possible.

Attention! Every time you give up alcohol you must get from your doctor drugs for the transition period between drinking alcohol and abstinence. Abrupt stop of drinking alcohol can be very dangerous for your health and even life.

***

Evening

- Repeat STOP (10 times every hour).
- Say slowly every 2 hours: sun, flower, seven, path, tee, run, yellow, apple, fish, rain, pen, water, smile, talk, life, sky.
- Small supper.
- Nice talk (no complaints) 30 min. When nobody to talk with, phone or internet conversation oral or written.
- Walk 20 min.
- Every time the desire to drink alcohol comes back to you, imagine that you want to continue without alcohol only a little bit more. Never think that you will never ever drink alcohol again. Of course this would be great but for some people it is impossible to stand the idea, especially at the beginning of the therapy. But instead of breaking the abstinence right away,

ALWAYS give yourself some time, even very short and say to yourself:

I will wait still one hour.

I will wait still 2 hours.

I will wait still 3 hours.

Etc.

I will wait still one day.

I will wait still 2 days.

I will wait still 3 days.

Etc.

Afer one hour or 2 hours or one day or 2 days passed by, ask yourself:

Do I feel the desire to drink alcohol?

No

In such a case you can continue with abstinence untill next time you feel the desire to drink alcohol.

Yes

In such a case you can make one more effort and one more time put untill later drinking alcohol again. Are you ready to make such an effort?

Yes

In this case you continue the abstinence.

No

In this case you are close to loose this time the battle with alcohol. This means you are not yet determined enough to continue the abstinence. Try again later and never think when giving up drinking alcohol that it is for always. Always think it is for as long as possible.

Attention! Every time you give up alcohol you must get from your doctor drugs for the transition period between drinking alcohol and abstinence. Abrupt stop of drinking alcohol can be very dangerous for your health and even life.

***

Night

Before sleep

- Take a shower (warm water) 1 min.
- Small physical excercise 3 min.

In Bed

- Repeat STOP (20 times)
- Say slowly untill you fall asleep: sun, flower, seven, path, tee, run, yellow, apple, fish, rain, pen, water, smile, talk, life, sky.

If you cannot fall asleep

- Say slowly untill you fall asleep: sun, flower, seven, path, tee, run, yellow, apple, fish, rain, pen, water, smile, talk, life, sky.

If above does not help

- Stand up and go to the toilet (when possible with as little light as possible)
- Say slowly untill you fall asleep: sun, flower, seven, path, tee, run, yellow, apple, fish, rain, pen, water, smile, talk, life, sky.

If above does not help

- Say STOP untill you fall asleep

If above does not help

- Go to the kitchen and have a very small snack.
- Back to the bed say slowly untill you fall asleep: sun, flower, seven, path, tee, run, yellow, apple, fish, rain, pen, water, smile, talk, life, sky.

If above does not help

- Say slowly untill morning: sun, flower, seven, path, tee, run, yellow, apple, fish, rain, pen, water, smile, talk, life, sky.

***

Day 2

Morning

* Repeat STOP (10 times every hour)

* Say slowly every 2 hours: sun, flower, seven, path, tee, run, yellow, apple, fish, rain, pen, water, smile, talk, life, sky.

* Small physical excercise (15 min)

* Small breakfast.

* Nice talk (no complaints) 25 min. When nobody to talk with, phone or internet conversation oral or written.

* Walk 20 min.

* Every time the desire to drink alcohol comes back to you, imagine that you want to continue without alcohol only a little bit more. Never think that you will never ever drink alcohol again. Of course this would be great but for some people it is impossible to stand the idea, especially at the beginning of the therapy. But instead of breaking the abstinence right away, ALWAYS give yourself some time, even very short and say to yourself:

I will wait still one hour.

I will wait still 2 hours.

I will wait still 3 hours.

Etc.

I will wait still one day.

I will wait still 2 days.

I will wait still 3 days.

Etc.

Afer one hour or 2 hours or one day or 2 days passed by, ask yourself:

Do I feel the desire to drink alcohol?

No

In such a case you can continue with abstinence untill next time you feel the desire to drink alcohol.

Yes

In such a case you can make one more effort and one more time put untill later drinking alcohol again. Are you ready to make such an effort?

Yes

In this case you continue the abstinence.

No

In this case you are close to loose this time the battle with alcohol. This means you are not yet determined enough to continue the abstinence.

Try again later and never think when giving up drinking alcohol that it is for always. Always think it is for as long as possible.

Attention! Every time you give up alcohol you must get from your doctor drugs for the transition period between drinking alcohol and abstinence. Abrupt stop of drinking alcohol can be very dangerous for your health and even life.

***

Afternoon

* Repeat STOP (10 times every hour.)

* Say slowly every 2 hours: sun, flower, seven, path, tee, run, yellow, apple, fish, rain, pen, water, smile, talk, life, sky.

* Dinner and half an hour break (you can sleep).

* Nice talk (no complaints) 30 min. When nobody to talk with, phone or internet conversation oral or written.

* Walk 20 min.

* Every time the desire to drink alcohol comes back to you, imagine that you want to continue without alcohol only a little bit more. Never think that you will never

ever drink alcohol again. Of course this would be great but for some people it is impossible to stand the idea, especially at the beginning of the therapy. But instead of breaking the abstinence right away, ALWAYS give yourself some time, even very short and say to yourself:

I will wait still one hour.

I will wait still 2 hours.

I will wait still 3 hours.

Etc.

I will wait still one day.

I will wait still 2 days.

I will wait still 3 days.

Etc.

Afer one hour or 2 hours or one day or 2 days passed by, ask yourself:

Do I feel the desire to drink alcohol?

No

In such a case you can continue with abstinence untill next time you feel the desire to drink alcohol.

Yes

In such a case you can make one more effort and one more time put untill later drinking alcohol again. Are you ready to make such an effort?

Yes

In this case you continue the abstinence.

No

In this case you are close to loose this time the battle with alcohol. This means you are not yet determined enough to continue the abstinence.

Try again later and never think when giving up drinking alcohol that it is for always. Always think it is for as long as possible.

Attention! Every time you give up alcohol you must get from your doctor drugs for the transition period between drinking alcohol and abstinence. Abrupt stop of drinking alcohol can be very dangerous for your health and even life.

***

Evening

- Repeat STOP (10 times every hour).
- Say slowly every 2 hours: sun, flower, seven, path, tee, run, yellow, apple, fish, rain, pen, water, smile, talk, life, sky.

- Small supper.
- Nice talk (no complaints) 30 min. When nobody to talk with, phone or internet conversation oral or written.
- Walk 20 min.
- Every time the desire to drink alcohol comes back to you, imagine that you want to continue without alcohol only a little bit more. Never think that you will never ever drink alcohol again. Of course this would be great but for some people it is impossible to stand the idea, especially at the beginning of the therapy. But instead of breaking the abstinence right away, ALWAYS give yourself some time, even very short and say to yourself:

  I will wait still one hour.

  I will wait still 2 hours.

  I will wait still 3 hours.

  Etc.

  I will wait still one day.

  I will wait still 2 days.

  I will wait still 3 days.

  Etc.

  Afer one hour or 2 hours or one day or 2 days passed by, ask yourself:

  Do I feel the desire to drink alcohol?

No

In such a case you can continue with abstinence untill next time you feel the desire to drink alcohol.

Yes

In such a case you can make one more effort and one more time put untill later drinking alcohol again. Are you ready to make such an effort?

Yes

In this case you continue the abstinence.

No

In this case you are close to loose this time the battle with alcohol. This means you are not yet determined enough to continue the abstinence. Try again later and never think when giving up drinking alcohol that it is for always. Always think it is for as long as possible.

Attention! Every time you give up alcohol you must get from your doctor drugs for the transition period between drinking alcohol and abstinence. Abrupt stop of drinking alcohol can be very dangerous for your health and even life.

***

Night

Before sleep

- Take a shower (warm water) 1 min.
- Small physical excercise 3 min.

In Bed

- Repeat STOP (20 times)
- Say slowly untill you fall asleep: sun, flower, seven, path, tee, run, yellow, apple, fish, rain, pen, water, smile, talk, life, sky.

If you cannot fall asleep

- Say slowly untill you fall asleep: sun, flower, seven, path, tee, run, yellow, apple, fish, rain, pen, water, smile, talk, life, sky.

If above does not help

- Stand up and go to the toilet (when possible with as little light as possible)
- Say slowly untill you fall asleep: sun, flower, seven, path, tee, run, yellow, apple, fish, rain, pen, water, smile, talk, life, sky.

If above does not help

- Say STOP untill you fall asleep

If above does not help

- Go to the kitchen and have a very small snack.

- Back to the bed say slowly untill you fall asleep: sun, flower, seven, path, tee, run, yellow, apple, fish, rain, pen, water, smile, talk, life, sky.

If above does not help

- Say slowly untill morning: sun, flower, seven, path, tee, run, yellow, apple, fish, rain, pen, water, smile, talk, life, sky.

***

Day 3

Morning

* Repeat STOP (10 times every hour)

* Say slowly every 2 hours: sun, flower, seven, path, tee, run, yellow, apple, fish, rain, pen, water, smile, talk, life, sky.

* Small physical excercise (15 min)

* Small breakfast.

* Nice talk (no complaints) 25 min. When nobody to talk with, phone or internet conversation oral or written.

* Walk 20 min.

* Every time the desire to drink alcohol comes back to you, imagine that you want to continue without alcohol

only a little bit more. Never think that you will never ever drink alcohol again. Of course this would be great but for some people it is impossible to stand the idea, especially at the beginning of the therapy. But instead of breaking the abstinence right away, ALWAYS give yourself some time, even very short and say to yourself:

I will wait still one hour.

I will wait still 2 hours.

I will wait still 3 hours.

Etc.

I will wait still one day.

I will wait still 2 days.

I will wait still 3 days.

Etc.

Afer one hour or 2 hours or one day or 2 days passed by, ask yourself:

Do I feel the desire to drink alcohol?

No

In such a case you can continue with abstinence untill next time you feel the desire to drink alcohol.

Yes

In such a case you can make one more effort and one more time put untill later drinking alcohol again. Are you ready to make such an effort?

Yes

In this case you continue the abstinence.

No

In this case you are close to loose this time the battle with alcohol. This means you are not yet determined enough to continue the abstinence.

Try again later and never think when giving up drinking alcohol that it is for always. Always think it is for as long as possible.

Attention! Every time you give up alcohol you must get from your doctor drugs for the transition period between drinking alcohol and abstinence. Abrupt stop of drinking alcohol can be very dangerous for your health and even life.

***

Afternoon

* Repeat STOP (10 times every hour.)

* Say slowly every 2 hours: sun, flower, seven, path, tee, run, yellow, apple, fish, rain, pen, water, smile, talk, life, sky.

* Dinner and half an hour break (you can sleep).

* Nice talk (no complaints) 30 min. When nobody to talk with, phone or internet conversation oral or written.

* Walk 20 min.

* Every time the desire to drink alcohol comes back to you, imagine that you want to continue without alcohol only a little bit more. Never think that you will never ever drink alcohol again. Of course this would be great but for some people it is impossible to stand the idea, especially at the beginning of the therapy. But instead of breaking the abstinence right away, ALWAYS give yourself some time, even very short and say to yourself:

I will wait still one hour.

I will wait still 2 hours.

I will wait still 3 hours.

Etc.

I will wait still one day.

I will wait still 2 days.

I will wait still 3 days.

Etc.

Afer one hour or 2 hours or one day or 2 days passed by, ask yourself:

Do I feel the desire to drink alcohol?

No

In such a case you can continue with abstinence untill next time you feel the desire to drink alcohol.

Yes

In such a case you can make one more effort and one more time put untill later drinking alcohol again. Are you ready to make such an effort?

Yes

In this case you continue the abstinence.

No

In this case you are close to loose this time the battle with alcohol. This means you are not yet determined enough to continue the abstinence.

Try again later and never think when giving up drinking alcohol that it is for always. Always think it is for as long as possible.

Attention! Every time you give up alcohol you must get from your doctor drugs for the transition period between drinking alcohol and abstinence. Abrupt stop of drinking alcohol can be very dangerous for your health and even life.

***

Evening

- Repeat STOP (10 times every hour).
- Say slowly every 2 hours: sun, flower, seven, path, tee, run, yellow, apple, fish, rain, pen, water, smile, talk, life, sky.
- Small supper.
- Nice talk (no complaints) 30 min. When nobody to talk with, phone or internet conversation oral or written.
- Walk 20 min.
- Every time the desire to drink alcohol comes back to you, imagine that you want to continue without alcohol only a little bit more. Never think that you will never ever drink alcohol again. Of course this would be great but for some people it is impossible to stand the idea, especially at the beginning of the therapy. But instead of breaking the abstinence right away,

ALWAYS give yourself some time, even very short and say to yourself:

I will wait still one hour.

I will wait still 2 hours.

I will wait still 3 hours.

Etc.

I will wait still one day.

I will wait still 2 days.

I will wait still 3 days.

Etc.

Afer one hour or 2 hours or one day or 2 days passed by, ask yourself:

Do I feel the desire to drink alcohol?

No

In such a case you can continue with abstinence untill next time you feel the desire to drink alcohol.

Yes

In such a case you can make one more effort and one more time put untill later drinking alcohol again. Are you ready to make such an effort?

Yes

In this case you continue the abstinence.

No

In this case you are close to loose this time the battle with alcohol. This means you are not yet determined enough to continue the abstinence. Try again later and never think when giving up drinking alcohol that it is for always. Always think it is for as long as possible.

Attention! Every time you give up alcohol you must get from your doctor drugs for the transition period between drinking alcohol and abstinence. Abrupt stop of drinking alcohol can be very dangerous for your health and even life.

***

Night

Before sleep

- Take a shower (warm water) 1 min.
- Small physical excercise 3 min.

In Bed

- Repeat STOP (20 times)
- Say slowly untill you fall asleep: sun, flower, seven, path, tee, run, yellow, apple, fish, rain, pen, water, smile, talk, life, sky.

If you cannot fall asleep

- Say slowly untill you fall asleep: sun, flower, seven, path, tee, run, yellow, apple, fish, rain, pen, water, smile, talk, life, sky.

If above does not help

- Stand up and go to the toilet (when possible with as little light as possible)
- Say slowly untill you fall asleep: sun, flower, seven, path, tee, run, yellow, apple, fish, rain, pen, water, smile, talk, life, sky.

If above does not help

- Say STOP untill you fall asleep

If above does not help

- Go to the kitchen and have a very small snack.
- Back to the bed say slowly untill you fall asleep: sun, flower, seven, path, tee, run, yellow, apple, fish, rain, pen, water, smile, talk, life, sky.

If above does not help

- Say slowly untill morning: sun, flower, seven, path, tee, run, yellow, apple, fish, rain, pen, water, smile, talk, life, sky.

***

Day 4

Morning

* Repeat STOP (10 times every hour)

* Say slowly every 2 hours: sun, flower, seven, path, tee, run, yellow, apple, fish, rain, pen, water, smile, talk, life, sky.

* Small physical excercise (15 min)

* Small breakfast.

* Nice talk (no complaints) 25 min. When nobody to talk with, phone or internet conversation oral or written.

* Walk 20 min.

* Every time the desire to drink alcohol comes back to you, imagine that you want to continue without alcohol only a little bit more. Never think that you will never ever drink alcohol again. Of course this would be great but for some people it is impossible to stand the idea, especially at the beginning of the therapy. But instead of breaking the abstinence right away, ALWAYS give yourself some time, even very short and say to yourself:

I will wait still one hour.

I will wait still 2 hours.

I will wait still 3 hours.

Etc.

I will wait still one day.

I will wait still 2 days.

I will wait still 3 days.

Etc.

Afer one hour or 2 hours or one day or 2 days passed by, ask yourself:

Do I feel the desire to drink alcohol?

No

In such a case you can continue with abstinence untill next time you feel the desire to drink alcohol.

Yes

In such a case you can make one more effort and one more time put untill later drinking alcohol again. Are you ready to make such an effort?

Yes

In this case you continue the abstinence.

No

In this case you are close to loose this time the battle with alcohol. This means you are not yet determined enough to continue the abstinence.

Try again later and never think when giving up drinking alcohol that it is for always. Always think it is for as long as possible.

Attention! Every time you give up alcohol you must get from your doctor drugs for the transition period between drinking alcohol and abstinence. Abrupt stop of drinking alcohol can be very dangerous for your health and even life.

***

Afternoon

* Repeat STOP (10 times every hour.)

* Say slowly every 2 hours: sun, flower, seven, path, tee, run, yellow, apple, fish, rain, pen, water, smile, talk, life, sky.

* Dinner and half an hour break (you can sleep).

* Nice talk (no complaints) 30 min. When nobody to talk with, phone or internet conversation oral or written.

* Walk 20 min.

* Every time the desire to drink alcohol comes back to you, imagine that you want to continue without alcohol only a little bit more. Never think that you will never

ever drink alcohol again. Of course this would be great but for some people it is impossible to stand the idea, especially at the beginning of the therapy. But instead of breaking the abstinence right away, ALWAYS give yourself some time, even very short and say to yourself:

I will wait still one hour.

I will wait still 2 hours.

I will wait still 3 hours.

Etc.

I will wait still one day.

I will wait still 2 days.

I will wait still 3 days.

Etc.

Afer one hour or 2 hours or one day or 2 days passed by, ask yourself:

Do I feel the desire to drink alcohol?

No

In such a case you can continue with abstinence untill next time you feel the desire to drink alcohol.

Yes

In such a case you can make one more effort and one more time put untill later drinking alcohol again. Are you ready to make such an effort?

Yes

In this case you continue the abstinence.

No

In this case you are close to loose this time the battle with alcohol. This means you are not yet determined enough to continue the abstinence.

Try again later and never think when giving up drinking alcohol that it is for always. Always think it is for as long as possible.

Attention! Every time you give up alcohol you must get from your doctor drugs for the transition period between drinking alcohol and abstinence. Abrupt stop of drinking alcohol can be very dangerous for your health and even life.

***

Evening

- Repeat STOP (10 times every hour).
- Say slowly every 2 hours: sun, flower, seven, path, tee, run, yellow, apple, fish, rain, pen, water, smile, talk, life, sky.

- Small supper.
- Nice talk (no complaints) 30 min. When nobody to talk with, phone or internet conversation oral or written.
- Walk 20 min.
- Every time the desire to drink alcohol comes back to you, imagine that you want to continue without alcohol only a little bit more. Never think that you will never ever drink alcohol again. Of course this would be great but for some people it is impossible to stand the idea, especially at the beginning of the therapy. But instead of breaking the abstinence right away, ALWAYS give yourself some time, even very short and say to yourself:

  I will wait still one hour.

  I will wait still 2 hours.

  I will wait still 3 hours.

  Etc.

  I will wait still one day.

  I will wait still 2 days.

  I will wait still 3 days.

  Etc.

  Afer one hour or 2 hours or one day or 2 days passed by, ask yourself:

  Do I feel the desire to drink alcohol?

No
In such a case you can continue with abstinence untill next time you feel the desire to drink alcohol.
Yes
In such a case you can make one more effort and one more time put untill later drinking alcohol again. Are you ready to make such an effort?
Yes
In this case you continue the abstinence.
No
In this case you are close to loose this time the battle with alcohol. This means you are not yet determined enough to continue the abstinence. Try again later and never think when giving up drinking alcohol that it is for always. Always think it is for as long as possible.
Attention! Every time you give up alcohol you must get from your doctor drugs for the transition period between drinking alcohol and abstinence. Abrupt stop of drinking alcohol can be very dangerous for your health and even life.

***

Night

Before sleep

- Take a shower (warm water) 1 min.
- Small physical excercise 3 min.

In Bed

- Repeat STOP (20 times)
- Say slowly untill you fall asleep: sun, flower, seven, path, tee, run, yellow, apple, fish, rain, pen, water, smile, talk, life, sky.

If you cannot fall asleep

- Say slowly untill you fall asleep: sun, flower, seven, path, tee, run, yellow, apple, fish, rain, pen, water, smile, talk, life, sky.

If above does not help

- Stand up and go to the toilet (when possible with as little light as possible)
- Say slowly untill you fall asleep: sun, flower, seven, path, tee, run, yellow, apple, fish, rain, pen, water, smile, talk, life, sky.

If above does not help

- Say STOP untill you fall asleep

If above does not help

- Go to the kitchen and have a very small snack.

- Back to the bed say slowly untill you fall asleep: sun, flower, seven, path, tee, run, yellow, apple, fish, rain, pen, water, smile, talk, life, sky.

If above does not help

- Say slowly untill morning: sun, flower, seven, path, tee, run, yellow, apple, fish, rain, pen, water, smile, talk, life, sky.

***

Day 5

Morning

* Repeat STOP (10 times every hour)

* Say slowly every 2 hours: sun, flower, seven, path, tee, run, yellow, apple, fish, rain, pen, water, smile, talk, life, sky.

* Small physical excercise (15 min)

* Small breakfast.

* Nice talk (no complaints) 25 min. When nobody to talk with, phone or internet conversation oral or written.

* Walk 20 min.

* Every time the desire to drink alcohol comes back to you, imagine that you want to continue without alcohol

only a little bit more. Never think that you will never ever drink alcohol again. Of course this would be great but for some people it is impossible to stand the idea, especially at the beginning of the therapy. But instead of breaking the abstinence right away, ALWAYS give yourself some time, even very short and say to yourself:

I will wait still one hour.

I will wait still 2 hours.

I will wait still 3 hours.

Etc.

I will wait still one day.

I will wait still 2 days.

I will wait still 3 days.

Etc.

Afer one hour or 2 hours or one day or 2 days passed by, ask yourself:

Do I feel the desire to drink alcohol?

No

In such a case you can continue with abstinence untill next time you feel the desire to drink alcohol.

Yes

In such a case you can make one more effort and one more time put untill later drinking alcohol again. Are you ready to make such an effort?

Yes

In this case you continue the abstinence.

No

In this case you are close to loose this time the battle with alcohol. This means you are not yet determined enough to continue the abstinence.

Try again later and never think when giving up drinking alcohol that it is for always. Always think it is for as long as possible.

Attention! Every time you give up alcohol you must get from your doctor drugs for the transition period between drinking alcohol and abstinence. Abrupt stop of drinking alcohol can be very dangerous for your health and even life.

***

Afternoon

* Repeat STOP (10 times every hour.)

* Say slowly every 2 hours: sun, flower, seven, path, tee, run, yellow, apple, fish, rain, pen, water, smile, talk, life, sky.

* Dinner and half an hour break (you can sleep).

* Nice talk (no complaints) 30 min. When nobody to talk with, phone or internet conversation oral or written.

* Walk 20 min.

* Every time the desire to drink alcohol comes back to you, imagine that you want to continue without alcohol only a little bit more. Never think that you will never ever drink alcohol again. Of course this would be great but for some people it is impossible to stand the idea, especially at the beginning of the therapy. But instead of breaking the abstinence right away, ALWAYS give yourself some time, even very short and say to yourself:

I will wait still one hour.

I will wait still 2 hours.

I will wait still 3 hours.

Etc.

I will wait still one day.

I will wait still 2 days.

I will wait still 3 days.

Etc.

Afer one hour or 2 hours or one day or 2 days passed by, ask yourself:

Do I feel the desire to drink alcohol?

No

In such a case you can continue with abstinence untill next time you feel the desire to drink alcohol.

Yes

In such a case you can make one more effort and one more time put untill later drinking alcohol again. Are you ready to make such an effort?

Yes

In this case you continue the abstinence.

No

In this case you are close to loose this time the battle with alcohol. This means you are not yet determined enough to continue the abstinence.

Try again later and never think when giving up drinking alcohol that it is for always. Always think it is for as long as possible.

Attention! Every time you give up alcohol you must get from your doctor drugs for the transition period between drinking alcohol and abstinence. Abrupt stop of drinking alcohol can be very dangerous for your health and even life.

***

Evening

- Repeat STOP (10 times every hour).
- Say slowly every 2 hours: sun, flower, seven, path, tee, run, yellow, apple, fish, rain, pen, water, smile, talk, life, sky.
- Small supper.
- Nice talk (no complaints) 30 min. When nobody to talk with, phone or internet conversation oral or written.
- Walk 20 min.
- Every time the desire to drink alcohol comes back to you, imagine that you want to continue without alcohol only a little bit more. Never think that you will never ever drink alcohol again. Of course this would be great but for some people it is impossible to stand the idea, especially at the beginning of the therapy. But instead of breaking the abstinence right away,

ALWAYS give yourself some time, even very short and say to yourself:

I will wait still one hour.

I will wait still 2 hours.

I will wait still 3 hours.

Etc.

I will wait still one day.

I will wait still 2 days.

I will wait still 3 days.

Etc.

Afer one hour or 2 hours or one day or 2 days passed by, ask yourself:

Do I feel the desire to drink alcohol?

No

In such a case you can continue with abstinence untill next time you feel the desire to drink alcohol.

Yes

In such a case you can make one more effort and one more time put untill later drinking alcohol again. Are you ready to make such an effort?

Yes

In this case you continue the abstinence.

No

In this case you are close to loose this time the battle with alcohol. This means you are not yet determined enough to continue the abstinence. Try again later and never think when giving up drinking alcohol that it is for always. Always think it is for as long as possible.

Attention! Every time you give up alcohol you must get from your doctor drugs for the transition period between drinking alcohol and abstinence. Abrupt stop of drinking alcohol can be very dangerous for your health and even life.

***

Night

Before sleep

- Take a shower (warm water) 1 min.
- Small physical excercise 3 min.

In Bed

- Repeat STOP (20 times)
- Say slowly untill you fall asleep: sun, flower, seven, path, tee, run, yellow, apple, fish, rain, pen, water, smile, talk, life, sky.

If you cannot fall asleep

- Say slowly untill you fall asleep: sun, flower, seven, path, tee, run, yellow, apple, fish, rain, pen, water, smile, talk, life, sky.

If above does not help

- Stand up and go to the toilet (when possible with as little light as possible)
- Say slowly untill you fall asleep: sun, flower, seven, path, tee, run, yellow, apple, fish, rain, pen, water, smile, talk, life, sky.

If above does not help

- Say STOP untill you fall asleep

If above does not help

- Go to the kitchen and have a very small snack.
- Back to the bed say slowly untill you fall asleep: sun, flower, seven, path, tee, run, yellow, apple, fish, rain, pen, water, smile, talk, life, sky.

If above does not help

- Say slowly untill morning: sun, flower, seven, path, tee, run, yellow, apple, fish, rain, pen, water, smile, talk, life, sky.

***

Day 6

Morning

* Repeat STOP (10 times every hour)

* Say slowly every 2 hours: sun, flower, seven, path, tee, run, yellow, apple, fish, rain, pen, water, smile, talk, life, sky.

* Small physical excercise (15 min)

* Small breakfast.

* Nice talk (no complaints) 25 min. When nobody to talk with, phone or internet conversation oral or written.

* Walk 20 min.

* Every time the desire to drink alcohol comes back to you, imagine that you want to continue without alcohol only a little bit more. Never think that you will never ever drink alcohol again. Of course this would be great but for some people it is impossible to stand the idea, especially at the beginning of the therapy. But instead of breaking the abstinence right away, ALWAYS give yourself some time, even very short and say to yourself:

I will wait still one hour.

I will wait still 2 hours.

I will wait still 3 hours.

Etc.

I will wait still one day.

I will wait still 2 days.

I will wait still 3 days.

Etc.

Afer one hour or 2 hours or one day or 2 days passed by, ask yourself:

Do I feel the desire to drink alcohol?

No

In such a case you can continue with abstinence untill next time you feel the desire to drink alcohol.

Yes

In such a case you can make one more effort and one more time put untill later drinking alcohol again. Are you ready to make such an effort?

Yes

In this case you continue the abstinence.

No

In this case you are close to loose this time the battle with alcohol. This means you are not yet determined enough to continue the abstinence.

Try again later and never think when giving up drinking alcohol that it is for always. Always think it is for as long as possible.

Attention! Every time you give up alcohol you must get from your doctor drugs for the transition period between drinking alcohol and abstinence. Abrupt stop of drinking alcohol can be very dangerous for your health and even life.

***

Afternoon

* Repeat STOP (10 times every hour.)

* Say slowly every 2 hours: sun, flower, seven, path, tee, run, yellow, apple, fish, rain, pen, water, smile, talk, life, sky.

* Dinner and half an hour break (you can sleep).

* Nice talk (no complaints) 30 min. When nobody to talk with, phone or internet conversation oral or written.

* Walk 20 min.

* Every time the desire to drink alcohol comes back to you, imagine that you want to continue without alcohol only a little bit more. Never think that you will never

ever drink alcohol again. Of course this would be great but for some people it is impossible to stand the idea, especially at the beginning of the therapy. But instead of breaking the abstinence right away, ALWAYS give yourself some time, even very short and say to yourself:

I will wait still one hour.

I will wait still 2 hours.

I will wait still 3 hours.

Etc.

I will wait still one day.

I will wait still 2 days.

I will wait still 3 days.

Etc.

Afer one hour or 2 hours or one day or 2 days passed by, ask yourself:

Do I feel the desire to drink alcohol?

No

In such a case you can continue with abstinence untill next time you feel the desire to drink alcohol.

Yes

In such a case you can make one more effort and one more time put untill later drinking alcohol again. Are you ready to make such an effort?

Yes

In this case you continue the abstinence.

No

In this case you are close to loose this time the battle with alcohol. This means you are not yet determined enough to continue the abstinence.

Try again later and never think when giving up drinking alcohol that it is for always. Always think it is for as long as possible.

Attention! Every time you give up alcohol you must get from your doctor drugs for the transition period between drinking alcohol and abstinence. Abrupt stop of drinking alcohol can be very dangerous for your health and even life.

***

Evening

- Repeat STOP (10 times every hour).
- Say slowly every 2 hours: sun, flower, seven, path, tee, run, yellow, apple, fish, rain, pen, water, smile, talk, life, sky.

- Small supper.
- Nice talk (no complaints) 30 min. When nobody to talk with, phone or internet conversation oral or written.
- Walk 20 min.
- Every time the desire to drink alcohol comes back to you, imagine that you want to continue without alcohol only a little bit more. Never think that you will never ever drink alcohol again. Of course this would be great but for some people it is impossible to stand the idea, especially at the beginning of the therapy. But instead of breaking the abstinence right away, ALWAYS give yourself some time, even very short and say to yourself:
  I will wait still one hour.
  I will wait still 2 hours.
  I will wait still 3 hours.
  Etc.
  I will wait still one day.
  I will wait still 2 days.
  I will wait still 3 days.
  Etc.
  Afer one hour or 2 hours or one day or 2 days passed by, ask yourself:
  Do I feel the desire to drink alcohol?

No

In such a case you can continue with abstinence untill next time you feel the desire to drink alcohol.

Yes

In such a case you can make one more effort and one more time put untill later drinking alcohol again. Are you ready to make such an effort?

Yes

In this case you continue the abstinence.

No

In this case you are close to loose this time the battle with alcohol. This means you are not yet determined enough to continue the abstinence. Try again later and never think when giving up drinking alcohol that it is for always. Always think it is for as long as possible.

Attention! Every time you give up alcohol you must get from your doctor drugs for the transition period between drinking alcohol and abstinence. Abrupt stop of drinking alcohol can be very dangerous for your health and even life.

***

Night

Before sleep

- Take a shower (warm water) 1 min.
- Small physical excercise 3 min.

In Bed

- Repeat STOP (20 times)
- Say slowly untill you fall asleep: sun, flower, seven, path, tee, run, yellow, apple, fish, rain, pen, water, smile, talk, life, sky.

If you cannot fall asleep

- Say slowly untill you fall asleep: sun, flower, seven, path, tee, run, yellow, apple, fish, rain, pen, water, smile, talk, life, sky.

If above does not help

- Stand up and go to the toilet (when possible with as little light as possible)
- Say slowly untill you fall asleep: sun, flower, seven, path, tee, run, yellow, apple, fish, rain, pen, water, smile, talk, life, sky.

If above does not help

- Say STOP untill you fall asleep

If above does not help

- Go to the kitchen and have a very small snack.

- Back to the bed say slowly untill you fall asleep: sun, flower, seven, path, tee, run, yellow, apple, fish, rain, pen, water, smile, talk, life, sky.

If above does not help

- Say slowly untill morning: sun, flower, seven, path, tee, run, yellow, apple, fish, rain, pen, water, smile, talk, life, sky.

***

Day 7

Morning

* Repeat STOP (10 times every hour)

* Say slowly every 2 hours: sun, flower, seven, path, tee, run, yellow, apple, fish, rain, pen, water, smile, talk, life, sky.

* Small physical excercise (15 min)

* Small breakfast.

* Nice talk (no complaints) 25 min. When nobody to talk with, phone or internet conversation oral or written.

* Walk 20 min.

* Every time the desire to drink alcohol comes back to you, imagine that you want to continue without alcohol

only a little bit more. Never think that you will never ever drink alcohol again. Of course this would be great but for some people it is impossible to stand the idea, especially at the beginning of the therapy. But instead of breaking the abstinence right away, ALWAYS give yourself some time, even very short and say to yourself:

I will wait still one hour.

I will wait still 2 hours.

I will wait still 3 hours.

Etc.

I will wait still one day.

I will wait still 2 days.

I will wait still 3 days.

Etc.

Afer one hour or 2 hours or one day or 2 days passed by, ask yourself:

Do I feel the desire to drink alcohol?

No

In such a case you can continue with abstinence untill next time you feel the desire to drink alcohol.

Yes

In such a case you can make one more effort and one more time put untill later drinking alcohol again. Are you ready to make such an effort?

Yes

In this case you continue the abstinence.

No

In this case you are close to loose this time the battle with alcohol. This means you are not yet determined enough to continue the abstinence.

Try again later and never think when giving up drinking alcohol that it is for always. Always think it is for as long as possible.

Attention! Every time you give up alcohol you must get from your doctor drugs for the transition period between drinking alcohol and abstinence. Abrupt stop of drinking alcohol can be very dangerous for your health and even life.

***

Afternoon

* Repeat STOP (10 times every hour.)

* Say slowly every 2 hours: sun, flower, seven, path, tee, run, yellow, apple, fish, rain, pen, water, smile, talk, life, sky.

* Dinner and half an hour break (you can sleep).

* Nice talk (no complaints) 30 min. When nobody to talk with, phone or internet conversation oral or written.

* Walk 20 min.

* Every time the desire to drink alcohol comes back to you, imagine that you want to continue without alcohol only a little bit more. Never think that you will never ever drink alcohol again. Of course this would be great but for some people it is impossible to stand the idea, especially at the beginning of the therapy. But instead of breaking the abstinence right away, ALWAYS give yourself some time, even very short and say to yourself:

I will wait still one hour.

I will wait still 2 hours.

I will wait still 3 hours.

Etc.

I will wait still one day.

I will wait still 2 days.

I will wait still 3 days.

Etc.

Afer one hour or 2 hours or one day or 2 days passed by, ask yourself:

Do I feel the desire to drink alcohol?

No

In such a case you can continue with abstinence untill next time you feel the desire to drink alcohol.

Yes

In such a case you can make one more effort and one more time put untill later drinking alcohol again. Are you ready to make such an effort?

Yes

In this case you continue the abstinence.

No

In this case you are close to loose this time the battle with alcohol. This means you are not yet determined enough to continue the abstinence.

Try again later and never think when giving up drinking alcohol that it is for always. Always think it is for as long as possible.

Attention! Every time you give up alcohol you must get from your doctor drugs for the transition period between drinking alcohol and abstinence. Abrupt stop of drinking alcohol can be very dangerous for your health and even life.

***

Evening

- Repeat STOP (10 times every hour).
- Say slowly every 2 hours: sun, flower, seven, path, tee, run, yellow, apple, fish, rain, pen, water, smile, talk, life, sky.
- Small supper.
- Nice talk (no complaints) 30 min. When nobody to talk with, phone or internet conversation oral or written.
- Walk 20 min.
- Every time the desire to drink alcohol comes back to you, imagine that you want to continue without alcohol only a little bit more. Never think that you will never ever drink alcohol again. Of course this would be great but for some people it is impossible to stand the idea, especially at the beginning of the therapy. But instead of breaking the abstinence right away,

ALWAYS give yourself some time, even very short and say to yourself:

I will wait still one hour.

I will wait still 2 hours.

I will wait still 3 hours.

Etc.

I will wait still one day.

I will wait still 2 days.

I will wait still 3 days.

Etc.

Afer one hour or 2 hours or one day or 2 days passed by, ask yourself:

Do I feel the desire to drink alcohol?

No

In such a case you can continue with abstinence untill next time you feel the desire to drink alcohol.

Yes

In such a case you can make one more effort and one more time put untill later drinking alcohol again. Are you ready to make such an effort?

Yes

In this case you continue the abstinence.

No

In this case you are close to loose this time the battle with alcohol. This means you are not yet determined enough to continue the abstinence. Try again later and never think when giving up drinking alcohol that it is for always. Always think it is for as long as possible.

Attention! Every time you give up alcohol you must get from your doctor drugs for the transition period between drinking alcohol and abstinence. Abrupt stop of drinking alcohol can be very dangerous for your health and even life.

***

Night

Before sleep

- Take a shower (warm water) 1 min.
- Small physical excercise 3 min.

In Bed

- Repeat STOP (20 times)
- Say slowly untill you fall asleep: sun, flower, seven, path, tee, run, yellow, apple, fish, rain, pen, water, smile, talk, life, sky.

If you cannot fall asleep

- Say slowly untill you fall asleep: sun, flower, seven, path, tee, run, yellow, apple, fish, rain, pen, water, smile, talk, life, sky.

If above does not help

- Stand up and go to the toilet (when possible with as little light as possible)
- Say slowly untill you fall asleep: sun, flower, seven, path, tee, run, yellow, apple, fish, rain, pen, water, smile, talk, life, sky.

If above does not help

- Say STOP untill you fall asleep

If above does not help

- Go to the kitchen and have a very small snack.
- Back to the bed say slowly untill you fall asleep: sun, flower, seven, path, tee, run, yellow, apple, fish, rain, pen, water, smile, talk, life, sky.

If above does not help

- Say slowly untill morning: sun, flower, seven, path, tee, run, yellow, apple, fish, rain, pen, water, smile, talk, life, sky.

***

Week Three

***

Day 1

Morning

* Repeat STOP (10 times every 2 hours)

* Say slowly every 3 hours: sun, flower, seven, path, tee, run, yellow, apple, fish, rain, pen, water, smile, talk, life, sky.

* Small physical excercise (20 min)

* Small breakfast.

* Nice talk (no complaints) 30 min. When nobody to talk with, phone or internet conversation oral or written.

* Walk 25 min.

* Every time the desire to drink alcohol comes back to you, imagine that you want to continue without alcohol only a little bit more. Never think that you will never ever drink alcohol again. Of course this would be great but for some people it is impossible to stand the idea, especially at the beginning of the therapy. But instead of breaking the abstinence right away, ALWAYS give yourself some time, even very short and say to yourself:

I will wait still one hour.

I will wait still 2 hours.

I will wait still 3 hours.

Etc.

I will wait still one day.

I will wait still 2 days.

I will wait still 3 days.

Etc.

Afer one hour or 2 hours or one day or 2 days passed by, ask yourself:

Do I feel the desire to drink alcohol?

No

In such a case you can continue with abstinence untill next time you feel the desire to drink alcohol.

Yes

In such a case you can make one more effort and one more time put untill later drinking alcohol again. Are you ready to make such an effort?

Yes

In this case you continue the abstinence.

No

In this case you are close to loose this time the battle with alcohol. This means you are not yet determined enough to continue the abstinence.

Try again later and never think when giving up drinking alcohol that it is for always. Always think it is for as long as possible.

Attention! Every time you give up alcohol you must get from your doctor drugs for the transition period between drinking alcohol and abstinence. Abrupt stop of drinking alcohol can be very dangerous for your health and even life.

***

Afternoon

* Repeat STOP (10 times every 2 hours).

* Say slowly every 3 hours: sun, flower, seven, path, tee, run, yellow, apple, fish, rain, pen, water, smile, talk, life, sky.

* Dinner and half an hour break (you can sleep).

* Nice talk (no complaints) 40 min. When nobody to talk with, phone or internet conversation oral or written.

* Walk 25 min.

* Every time the desire to drink alcohol comes back to you, imagine that you want to continue without alcohol only a little bit more. Never think that you will never

ever drink alcohol again. Of course this would be great but for some people it is impossible to stand the idea, especially at the beginning of the therapy. But instead of breaking the abstinence right away, ALWAYS give yourself some time, even very short and say to yourself:

I will wait still one hour.

I will wait still 2 hours.

I will wait still 3 hours.

Etc.

I will wait still one day.

I will wait still 2 days.

I will wait still 3 days.

Etc.

Afer one hour or 2 hours or one day or 2 days passed by, ask yourself:

Do I feel the desire to drink alcohol?

No

In such a case you can continue with abstinence untill next time you feel the desire to drink alcohol.

Yes

In such a case you can make one more effort and one more time put untill later drinking alcohol again. Are you ready to make such an effort?

Yes

In this case you continue the abstinence.

No

In this case you are close to loose this time the battle with alcohol. This means you are not yet determined enough to continue the abstinence.

Try again later and never think when giving up drinking alcohol that it is for always. Always think it is for as long as possible.

Attention! Every time you give up alcohol you must get from your doctor drugs for the transition period between drinking alcohol and abstinence. Abrupt stop of drinking alcohol can be very dangerous for your health and even life.

***

Evening

- Repeat STOP (10 times every 2 hours).
- Say slowly every 3 hours: sun, flower, seven, path, tee, run, yellow, apple, fish, rain, pen, water, smile, talk, life, sky.

- Small supper.
- Nice talk (no complaints) 40 min. When nobody to talk with, phone or internet conversation oral or written.
- Walk 25 min.
- Every time the desire to drink alcohol comes back to you, imagine that you want to continue without alcohol only a little bit more. Never think that you will never ever drink alcohol again. Of course this would be great but for some people it is impossible to stand the idea, especially at the beginning of the therapy. But instead of breaking the abstinence right away, ALWAYS give yourself some time, even very short and say to yourself:
  I will wait still one hour.
  I will wait still 2 hours.
  I will wait still 3 hours.
  Etc.
  I will wait still one day.
  I will wait still 2 days.
  I will wait still 3 days.
  Etc.
  Afer one hour or 2 hours or one day or 2 days passed by, ask yourself:
  Do I feel the desire to drink alcohol?

No

In such a case you can continue with abstinence untill next time you feel the desire to drink alcohol.

Yes

In such a case you can make one more effort and one more time put untill later drinking alcohol again. Are you ready to make such an effort?

Yes

In this case you continue the abstinence.

No

In this case you are close to loose this time the battle with alcohol. This means you are not yet determined enough to continue the abstinence. Try again later and never think when giving up drinking alcohol that it is for always. Always think it is for as long as possible.

Attention! Every time you give up alcohol you must get from your doctor drugs for the transition period between drinking alcohol and abstinence. Abrupt stop of drinking alcohol can be very dangerous for your health and even life.

***

Night

Before sleep

- Take a shower (warm water) 1 min.
- Small physical excercise 3 min.

In Bed

- Repeat STOP (20 times)
- Say slowly untill you fall asleep: sun, flower, seven, path, tee, run, yellow, apple, fish, rain, pen, water, smile, talk, life, sky.

If you cannot fall asleep

- Say slowly untill you fall asleep: sun, flower, seven, path, tee, run, yellow, apple, fish, rain, pen, water, smile, talk, life, sky.

If above does not help

- Stand up and go to the toilet (when possible with as little light as possible)
- Say slowly untill you fall asleep: sun, flower, seven, path, tee, run, yellow, apple, fish, rain, pen, water, smile, talk, life, sky.

If above does not help

- Say STOP untill you fall asleep

If above does not help

- Go to the kitchen and have a very small snack.

- Back to the bed say slowly untill you fall asleep: sun, flower, seven, path, tee, run, yellow, apple, fish, rain, pen, water, smile, talk, life, sky.

If above does not help

- Say slowly untill morning: sun, flower, seven, path, tee, run, yellow, apple, fish, rain, pen, water, smile, talk, life, sky.

***

Day 2

Morning

* Repeat STOP (10 times every 2 hours)

* Say slowly every 3 hours: sun, flower, seven, path, tee, run, yellow, apple, fish, rain, pen, water, smile, talk, life, sky.

* Small physical excercise (20 min)

* Small breakfast.

* Nice talk (no complaints) 30 min. When nobody to talk with, phone or internet conversation oral or written.

* Walk 25 min.

* Every time the desire to drink alcohol comes back to you, imagine that you want to continue without alcohol

only a little bit more. Never think that you will never ever drink alcohol again. Of course this would be great but for some people it is impossible to stand the idea, especially at the beginning of the therapy. But instead of breaking the abstinence right away, ALWAYS give yourself some time, even very short and say to yourself:

I will wait still one hour.

I will wait still 2 hours.

I will wait still 3 hours.

Etc.

I will wait still one day.

I will wait still 2 days.

I will wait still 3 days.

Etc.

Afer one hour or 2 hours or one day or 2 days passed by, ask yourself:

Do I feel the desire to drink alcohol?

No

In such a case you can continue with abstinence untill next time you feel the desire to drink alcohol.

Yes

In such a case you can make one more effort and one more time put untill later drinking alcohol again. Are you ready to make such an effort?

Yes

In this case you continue the abstinence.

No

In this case you are close to loose this time the battle with alcohol. This means you are not yet determined enough to continue the abstinence.

Try again later and never think when giving up drinking alcohol that it is for always. Always think it is for as long as possible.

Attention! Every time you give up alcohol you must get from your doctor drugs for the transition period between drinking alcohol and abstinence. Abrupt stop of drinking alcohol can be very dangerous for your health and even life.

***

Afternoon

* Repeat STOP (10 times every 2 hours).

* Say slowly every 3 hours: sun, flower, seven, path, tee, run, yellow, apple, fish, rain, pen, water, smile, talk, life, sky.

* Dinner and half an hour break (you can sleep).

* Nice talk (no complaints) 40 min. When nobody to talk with, phone or internet conversation oral or written.

* Walk 25 min.

* Every time the desire to drink alcohol comes back to you, imagine that you want to continue without alcohol only a little bit more. Never think that you will never ever drink alcohol again. Of course this would be great but for some people it is impossible to stand the idea, especially at the beginning of the therapy. But instead of breaking the abstinence right away, ALWAYS give yourself some time, even very short and say to yourself:

I will wait still one hour.

I will wait still 2 hours.

I will wait still 3 hours.

Etc.

I will wait still one day.

I will wait still 2 days.

I will wait still 3 days.

Etc.

Afer one hour or 2 hours or one day or 2 days passed by, ask yourself:

Do I feel the desire to drink alcohol?

No

In such a case you can continue with abstinence untill next time you feel the desire to drink alcohol.

Yes

In such a case you can make one more effort and one more time put untill later drinking alcohol again. Are you ready to make such an effort?

Yes

In this case you continue the abstinence.

No

In this case you are close to loose this time the battle with alcohol. This means you are not yet determined enough to continue the abstinence.

Try again later and never think when giving up drinking alcohol that it is for always. Always think it is for as long as possible.

Attention! Every time you give up alcohol you must get from your doctor drugs for the transition period between drinking alcohol and abstinence. Abrupt stop of drinking alcohol can be very dangerous for your health and even life.

***

Evening

- Repeat STOP (10 times every 2 hours).
- Say slowly every 3 hours: sun, flower, seven, path, tee, run, yellow, apple, fish, rain, pen, water, smile, talk, life, sky.
- Small supper.
- Nice talk (no complaints) 40 min. When nobody to talk with, phone or internet conversation oral or written.
- Walk 25 min.
- Every time the desire to drink alcohol comes back to you, imagine that you want to continue without alcohol only a little bit more. Never think that you will never ever drink alcohol again. Of course this would be great but for some people it is impossible to stand the idea, especially at the beginning of the therapy. But instead of breaking the abstinence right away,

ALWAYS give yourself some time, even very short and say to yourself:

I will wait still one hour.

I will wait still 2 hours.

I will wait still 3 hours.

Etc.

I will wait still one day.

I will wait still 2 days.

I will wait still 3 days.

Etc.

Afer one hour or 2 hours or one day or 2 days passed by, ask yourself:

Do I feel the desire to drink alcohol?

No

In such a case you can continue with abstinence untill next time you feel the desire to drink alcohol.

Yes

In such a case you can make one more effort and one more time put untill later drinking alcohol again. Are you ready to make such an effort?

Yes

In this case you continue the abstinence.

No

In this case you are close to loose this time the battle with alcohol. This means you are not yet determined enough to continue the abstinence. Try again later and never think when giving up drinking alcohol that it is for always. Always think it is for as long as possible.

Attention! Every time you give up alcohol you must get from your doctor drugs for the transition period between drinking alcohol and abstinence. Abrupt stop of drinking alcohol can be very dangerous for your health and even life.

***

Night

Before sleep

- Take a shower (warm water) 1 min.
- Small physical excercise 3 min.

In Bed

- Repeat STOP (20 times)
- Say slowly untill you fall asleep: sun, flower, seven, path, tee, run, yellow, apple, fish, rain, pen, water, smile, talk, life, sky.

If you cannot fall asleep

- Say slowly untill you fall asleep: sun, flower, seven, path, tee, run, yellow, apple, fish, rain, pen, water, smile, talk, life, sky.

If above does not help

- Stand up and go to the toilet (when possible with as little light as possible)
- Say slowly untill you fall asleep: sun, flower, seven, path, tee, run, yellow, apple, fish, rain, pen, water, smile, talk, life, sky.

If above does not help

- Say STOP untill you fall asleep

If above does not help

- Go to the kitchen and have a very small snack.
- Back to the bed say slowly untill you fall asleep: sun, flower, seven, path, tee, run, yellow, apple, fish, rain, pen, water, smile, talk, life, sky.

If above does not help

- Say slowly untill morning: sun, flower, seven, path, tee, run, yellow, apple, fish, rain, pen, water, smile, talk, life, sky.

***

Day 3

Morning

* Repeat STOP (10 times every 2 hours)

* Say slowly every 3 hours: sun, flower, seven, path, tee, run, yellow, apple, fish, rain, pen, water, smile, talk, life, sky.

* Small physical excercise (20 min)

* Small breakfast.

* Nice talk (no complaints) 30 min. When nobody to talk with, phone or internet conversation oral or written.

* Walk 25 min.

* Every time the desire to drink alcohol comes back to you, imagine that you want to continue without alcohol only a little bit more. Never think that you will never ever drink alcohol again. Of course this would be great but for some people it is impossible to stand the idea, especially at the beginning of the therapy. But instead of breaking the abstinence right away, ALWAYS give yourself some time, even very short and say to yourself:

I will wait still one hour.

I will wait still 2 hours.

I will wait still 3 hours.

Etc.

I will wait still one day.

I will wait still 2 days.

I will wait still 3 days.

Etc.

Afer one hour or 2 hours or one day or 2 days passed by, ask yourself:

Do I feel the desire to drink alcohol?

No

In such a case you can continue with abstinence untill next time you feel the desire to drink alcohol.

Yes

In such a case you can make one more effort and one more time put untill later drinking alcohol again. Are you ready to make such an effort?

Yes

In this case you continue the abstinence.

No

In this case you are close to loose this time the battle with alcohol. This means you are not yet determined enough to continue the abstinence.

Try again later and never think when giving up drinking alcohol that it is for always. Always think it is for as long as possible.

Attention! Every time you give up alcohol you must get from your doctor drugs for the transition period between drinking alcohol and abstinence. Abrupt stop of drinking alcohol can be very dangerous for your health and even life.

***

Afternoon

* Repeat STOP (10 times every 2 hours).

* Say slowly every 3 hours: sun, flower, seven, path, tee, run, yellow, apple, fish, rain, pen, water, smile, talk, life, sky.

* Dinner and half an hour break (you can sleep).

* Nice talk (no complaints) 40 min. When nobody to talk with, phone or internet conversation oral or written.

* Walk 25 min.

* Every time the desire to drink alcohol comes back to you, imagine that you want to continue without alcohol only a little bit more. Never think that you will never

ever drink alcohol again. Of course this would be great but for some people it is impossible to stand the idea, especially at the beginning of the therapy. But instead of breaking the abstinence right away, ALWAYS give yourself some time, even very short and say to yourself:

I will wait still one hour.

I will wait still 2 hours.

I will wait still 3 hours.

Etc.

I will wait still one day.

I will wait still 2 days.

I will wait still 3 days.

Etc.

Afer one hour or 2 hours or one day or 2 days passed by, ask yourself:

Do I feel the desire to drink alcohol?

No

In such a case you can continue with abstinence untill next time you feel the desire to drink alcohol.

Yes

In such a case you can make one more effort and one more time put untill later drinking alcohol again. Are you ready to make such an effort?

Yes

In this case you continue the abstinence.

No

In this case you are close to loose this time the battle with alcohol. This means you are not yet determined enough to continue the abstinence.

Try again later and never think when giving up drinking alcohol that it is for always. Always think it is for as long as possible.

Attention! Every time you give up alcohol you must get from your doctor drugs for the transition period between drinking alcohol and abstinence. Abrupt stop of drinking alcohol can be very dangerous for your health and even life.

***

Evening

- Repeat STOP (10 times every 2 hours).
- Say slowly every 3 hours: sun, flower, seven, path, tee, run, yellow, apple, fish, rain, pen, water, smile, talk, life, sky.

- Small supper.
- Nice talk (no complaints) 40 min. When nobody to talk with, phone or internet conversation oral or written.
- Walk 25 min.
- Every time the desire to drink alcohol comes back to you, imagine that you want to continue without alcohol only a little bit more. Never think that you will never ever drink alcohol again. Of course this would be great but for some people it is impossible to stand the idea, especially at the beginning of the therapy. But instead of breaking the abstinence right away, ALWAYS give yourself some time, even very short and say to yourself:
I will wait still one hour.
I will wait still 2 hours.
I will wait still 3 hours.
Etc.
I will wait still one day.
I will wait still 2 days.
I will wait still 3 days.
Etc.
Afer one hour or 2 hours or one day or 2 days passed by, ask yourself:
Do I feel the desire to drink alcohol?

No

In such a case you can continue with abstinence untill next time you feel the desire to drink alcohol.

Yes

In such a case you can make one more effort and one more time put untill later drinking alcohol again. Are you ready to make such an effort?

Yes

In this case you continue the abstinence.

No

In this case you are close to loose this time the battle with alcohol. This means you are not yet determined enough to continue the abstinence. Try again later and never think when giving up drinking alcohol that it is for always. Always think it is for as long as possible.

Attention! Every time you give up alcohol you must get from your doctor drugs for the transition period between drinking alcohol and abstinence. Abrupt stop of drinking alcohol can be very dangerous for your health and even life.

***

Night

Before sleep

- Take a shower (warm water) 1 min.
- Small physical excercise 3 min.

In Bed

- Repeat STOP (20 times)
- Say slowly untill you fall asleep: sun, flower, seven, path, tee, run, yellow, apple, fish, rain, pen, water, smile, talk, life, sky.

If you cannot fall asleep

- Say slowly untill you fall asleep: sun, flower, seven, path, tee, run, yellow, apple, fish, rain, pen, water, smile, talk, life, sky.

If above does not help

- Stand up and go to the toilet (when possible with as little light as possible)
- Say slowly untill you fall asleep: sun, flower, seven, path, tee, run, yellow, apple, fish, rain, pen, water, smile, talk, life, sky.

If above does not help

- Say STOP untill you fall asleep

If above does not help

- Go to the kitchen and have a very small snack.

- Back to the bed say slowly untill you fall asleep: sun, flower, seven, path, tee, run, yellow, apple, fish, rain, pen, water, smile, talk, life, sky.

If above does not help

- Say slowly untill morning: sun, flower, seven, path, tee, run, yellow, apple, fish, rain, pen, water, smile, talk, life, sky.

***

Day 4

Morning

* Repeat STOP (10 times every 2 hours)

* Say slowly every 3 hours: sun, flower, seven, path, tee, run, yellow, apple, fish, rain, pen, water, smile, talk, life, sky.

* Small physical excercise (20 min)

* Small breakfast.

* Nice talk (no complaints) 30 min. When nobody to talk with, phone or internet conversation oral or written.

* Walk 25 min.

* Every time the desire to drink alcohol comes back to you, imagine that you want to continue without alcohol

only a little bit more. Never think that you will never ever drink alcohol again. Of course this would be great but for some people it is impossible to stand the idea, especially at the beginning of the therapy. But instead of breaking the abstinence right away, ALWAYS give yourself some time, even very short and say to yourself:

I will wait still one hour.

I will wait still 2 hours.

I will wait still 3 hours.

Etc.

I will wait still one day.

I will wait still 2 days.

I will wait still 3 days.

Etc.

Afer one hour or 2 hours or one day or 2 days passed by, ask yourself:

Do I feel the desire to drink alcohol?

No

In such a case you can continue with abstinence untill next time you feel the desire to drink alcohol.

Yes

In such a case you can make one more effort and one more time put untill later drinking alcohol again. Are you ready to make such an effort?

Yes

In this case you continue the abstinence.

No

In this case you are close to loose this time the battle with alcohol. This means you are not yet determined enough to continue the abstinence.

Try again later and never think when giving up drinking alcohol that it is for always. Always think it is for as long as possible.

Attention! Every time you give up alcohol you must get from your doctor drugs for the transition period between drinking alcohol and abstinence. Abrupt stop of drinking alcohol can be very dangerous for your health and even life.

***

Afternoon

* Repeat STOP (10 times every 2 hours).

* Say slowly every 3 hours: sun, flower, seven, path, tee, run, yellow, apple, fish, rain, pen, water, smile, talk, life, sky.

* Dinner and half an hour break (you can sleep).

* Nice talk (no complaints) 40 min. When nobody to talk with, phone or internet conversation oral or written.

* Walk 25 min.

* Every time the desire to drink alcohol comes back to you, imagine that you want to continue without alcohol only a little bit more. Never think that you will never ever drink alcohol again. Of course this would be great but for some people it is impossible to stand the idea, especially at the beginning of the therapy. But instead of breaking the abstinence right away, ALWAYS give yourself some time, even very short and say to yourself:

I will wait still one hour.

I will wait still 2 hours.

I will wait still 3 hours.

Etc.

I will wait still one day.

I will wait still 2 days.

I will wait still 3 days.

Etc.

Afer one hour or 2 hours or one day or 2 days passed by, ask yourself:

Do I feel the desire to drink alcohol?

No

In such a case you can continue with abstinence untill next time you feel the desire to drink alcohol.

Yes

In such a case you can make one more effort and one more time put untill later drinking alcohol again. Are you ready to make such an effort?

Yes

In this case you continue the abstinence.

No

In this case you are close to loose this time the battle with alcohol. This means you are not yet determined enough to continue the abstinence.

Try again later and never think when giving up drinking alcohol that it is for always. Always think it is for as long as possible.

Attention! Every time you give up alcohol you must get from your doctor drugs for the transition period between drinking alcohol and abstinence. Abrupt stop of drinking alcohol can be very dangerous for your health and even life.

***

Evening

- Repeat STOP (10 times every 2 hours).
- Say slowly every 3 hours: sun, flower, seven, path, tee, run, yellow, apple, fish, rain, pen, water, smile, talk, life, sky.
- Small supper.
- Nice talk (no complaints) 40 min. When nobody to talk with, phone or internet conversation oral or written.
- Walk 25 min.
- Every time the desire to drink alcohol comes back to you, imagine that you want to continue without alcohol only a little bit more. Never think that you will never ever drink alcohol again. Of course this would be great but for some people it is impossible to stand the idea, especially at the beginning of the therapy. But instead of breaking the abstinence right away,

ALWAYS give yourself some time, even very short and say to yourself:

I will wait still one hour.

I will wait still 2 hours.

I will wait still 3 hours.

Etc.

I will wait still one day.

I will wait still 2 days.

I will wait still 3 days.

Etc.

Afer one hour or 2 hours or one day or 2 days passed by, ask yourself:

Do I feel the desire to drink alcohol?

No

In such a case you can continue with abstinence untill next time you feel the desire to drink alcohol.

Yes

In such a case you can make one more effort and one more time put untill later drinking alcohol again. Are you ready to make such an effort?

Yes

In this case you continue the abstinence.

No

In this case you are close to loose this time the battle with alcohol. This means you are not yet determined enough to continue the abstinence. Try again later and never think when giving up drinking alcohol that it is for always. Always think it is for as long as possible.

Attention! Every time you give up alcohol you must get from your doctor drugs for the transition period between drinking alcohol and abstinence. Abrupt stop of drinking alcohol can be very dangerous for your health and even life.

***

Night

Before sleep

- Take a shower (warm water) 1 min.
- Small physical excercise 3 min.

In Bed

- Repeat STOP (20 times)
- Say slowly untill you fall asleep: sun, flower, seven, path, tee, run, yellow, apple, fish, rain, pen, water, smile, talk, life, sky.

If you cannot fall asleep

- Say slowly untill you fall asleep: sun, flower, seven, path, tee, run, yellow, apple, fish, rain, pen, water, smile, talk, life, sky.

If above does not help

- Stand up and go to the toilet (when possible with as little light as possible)
- Say slowly untill you fall asleep: sun, flower, seven, path, tee, run, yellow, apple, fish, rain, pen, water, smile, talk, life, sky.

If above does not help

- Say STOP untill you fall asleep

If above does not help

- Go to the kitchen and have a very small snack.
- Back to the bed say slowly untill you fall asleep: sun, flower, seven, path, tee, run, yellow, apple, fish, rain, pen, water, smile, talk, life, sky.

If above does not help

- Say slowly untill morning: sun, flower, seven, path, tee, run, yellow, apple, fish, rain, pen, water, smile, talk, life, sky.

***

Day 5

Morning

* Repeat STOP (10 times every 2 hours)

* Say slowly every 3 hours: sun, flower, seven, path, tee, run, yellow, apple, fish, rain, pen, water, smile, talk, life, sky.

* Small physical excercise (20 min)

* Small breakfast.

* Nice talk (no complaints) 30 min. When nobody to talk with, phone or internet conversation oral or written.

* Walk 25 min.

* Every time the desire to drink alcohol comes back to you, imagine that you want to continue without alcohol only a little bit more. Never think that you will never ever drink alcohol again. Of course this would be great but for some people it is impossible to stand the idea, especially at the beginning of the therapy. But instead of breaking the abstinence right away, ALWAYS give yourself some time, even very short and say to yourself:

I will wait still one hour.

I will wait still 2 hours.

I will wait still 3 hours.

Etc.

I will wait still one day.

I will wait still 2 days.

I will wait still 3 days.

Etc.

Afer one hour or 2 hours or one day or 2 days passed by, ask yourself:

Do I feel the desire to drink alcohol?

No

In such a case you can continue with abstinence untill next time you feel the desire to drink alcohol.

Yes

In such a case you can make one more effort and one more time put untill later drinking alcohol again. Are you ready to make such an effort?

Yes

In this case you continue the abstinence.

No

In this case you are close to loose this time the battle with alcohol. This means you are not yet determined enough to continue the abstinence.

Try again later and never think when giving up drinking alcohol that it is for always. Always think it is for as long as possible.

Attention! Every time you give up alcohol you must get from your doctor drugs for the transition period between drinking alcohol and abstinence. Abrupt stop of drinking alcohol can be very dangerous for your health and even life.

***

Afternoon

* Repeat STOP (10 times every 2 hours).

* Say slowly every 3 hours: sun, flower, seven, path, tee, run, yellow, apple, fish, rain, pen, water, smile, talk, life, sky.

* Dinner and half an hour break (you can sleep).

* Nice talk (no complaints) 40 min. When nobody to talk with, phone or internet conversation oral or written.

* Walk 25 min.

* Every time the desire to drink alcohol comes back to you, imagine that you want to continue without alcohol only a little bit more. Never think that you will never

ever drink alcohol again. Of course this would be great but for some people it is impossible to stand the idea, especially at the beginning of the therapy. But instead of breaking the abstinence right away, ALWAYS give yourself some time, even very short and say to yourself:

I will wait still one hour.

I will wait still 2 hours.

I will wait still 3 hours.

Etc.

I will wait still one day.

I will wait still 2 days.

I will wait still 3 days.

Etc.

Afer one hour or 2 hours or one day or 2 days passed by, ask yourself:

Do I feel the desire to drink alcohol?

No

In such a case you can continue with abstinence untill next time you feel the desire to drink alcohol.

Yes

In such a case you can make one more effort and one more time put untill later drinking alcohol again. Are you ready to make such an effort?

Yes

In this case you continue the abstinence.

No

In this case you are close to loose this time the battle with alcohol. This means you are not yet determined enough to continue the abstinence.

Try again later and never think when giving up drinking alcohol that it is for always. Always think it is for as long as possible.

Attention! Every time you give up alcohol you must get from your doctor drugs for the transition period between drinking alcohol and abstinence. Abrupt stop of drinking alcohol can be very dangerous for your health and even life.

***

Evening

- Repeat STOP (10 times every 2 hours).
- Say slowly every 3 hours: sun, flower, seven, path, tee, run, yellow, apple, fish, rain, pen, water, smile, talk, life, sky.

- Small supper.
- Nice talk (no complaints) 40 min. When nobody to talk with, phone or internet conversation oral or written.
- Walk 25 min.
- Every time the desire to drink alcohol comes back to you, imagine that you want to continue without alcohol only a little bit more. Never think that you will never ever drink alcohol again. Of course this would be great but for some people it is impossible to stand the idea, especially at the beginning of the therapy. But instead of breaking the abstinence right away, ALWAYS give yourself some time, even very short and say to yourself:
  I will wait still one hour.
  I will wait still 2 hours.
  I will wait still 3 hours.
  Etc.
  I will wait still one day.
  I will wait still 2 days.
  I will wait still 3 days.
  Etc.
  Afer one hour or 2 hours or one day or 2 days passed by, ask yourself:
  Do I feel the desire to drink alcohol?

No

In such a case you can continue with abstinence untill next time you feel the desire to drink alcohol.

Yes

In such a case you can make one more effort and one more time put untill later drinking alcohol again. Are you ready to make such an effort?

Yes

In this case you continue the abstinence.

No

In this case you are close to loose this time the battle with alcohol. This means you are not yet determined enough to continue the abstinence. Try again later and never think when giving up drinking alcohol that it is for always. Always think it is for as long as possible.

Attention! Every time you give up alcohol you must get from your doctor drugs for the transition period between drinking alcohol and abstinence. Abrupt stop of drinking alcohol can be very dangerous for your health and even life.

***

Night

Before sleep

- Take a shower (warm water) 1 min.
- Small physical excercise 3 min.

In Bed

- Repeat STOP (20 times)
- Say slowly untill you fall asleep: sun, flower, seven, path, tee, run, yellow, apple, fish, rain, pen, water, smile, talk, life, sky.

If you cannot fall asleep

- Say slowly untill you fall asleep: sun, flower, seven, path, tee, run, yellow, apple, fish, rain, pen, water, smile, talk, life, sky.

If above does not help

- Stand up and go to the toilet (when possible with as little light as possible)
- Say slowly untill you fall asleep: sun, flower, seven, path, tee, run, yellow, apple, fish, rain, pen, water, smile, talk, life, sky.

If above does not help

- Say STOP untill you fall asleep

If above does not help

- Go to the kitchen and have a very small snack.

- Back to the bed say slowly untill you fall asleep: sun, flower, seven, path, tee, run, yellow, apple, fish, rain, pen, water, smile, talk, life, sky.

If above does not help

- Say slowly untill morning: sun, flower, seven, path, tee, run, yellow, apple, fish, rain, pen, water, smile, talk, life, sky.

***

Day 6

Morning

* Repeat STOP (10 times every 2 hours)

* Say slowly every 3 hours: sun, flower, seven, path, tee, run, yellow, apple, fish, rain, pen, water, smile, talk, life, sky.

* Small physical excercise (20 min)

* Small breakfast.

* Nice talk (no complaints) 30 min. When nobody to talk with, phone or internet conversation oral or written.

* Walk 25 min.

* Every time the desire to drink alcohol comes back to you, imagine that you want to continue without alcohol

only a little bit more. Never think that you will never ever drink alcohol again. Of course this would be great but for some people it is impossible to stand the idea, especially at the beginning of the therapy. But instead of breaking the abstinence right away, ALWAYS give yourself some time, even very short and say to yourself:

I will wait still one hour.

I will wait still 2 hours.

I will wait still 3 hours.

Etc.

I will wait still one day.

I will wait still 2 days.

I will wait still 3 days.

Etc.

Afer one hour or 2 hours or one day or 2 days passed by, ask yourself:

Do I feel the desire to drink alcohol?

No

In such a case you can continue with abstinence untill next time you feel the desire to drink alcohol.

Yes

In such a case you can make one more effort and one more time put untill later drinking alcohol again. Are you ready to make such an effort?

Yes

In this case you continue the abstinence.

No

In this case you are close to loose this time the battle with alcohol. This means you are not yet determined enough to continue the abstinence.

Try again later and never think when giving up drinking alcohol that it is for always. Always think it is for as long as possible.

Attention! Every time you give up alcohol you must get from your doctor drugs for the transition period between drinking alcohol and abstinence. Abrupt stop of drinking alcohol can be very dangerous for your health and even life.

***

Afternoon

* Repeat STOP (10 times every 2 hours).

* Say slowly every 3 hours: sun, flower, seven, path, tee, run, yellow, apple, fish, rain, pen, water, smile, talk, life, sky.

* Dinner and half an hour break (you can sleep).

* Nice talk (no complaints) 40 min. When nobody to talk with, phone or internet conversation oral or written.

* Walk 25 min.

* Every time the desire to drink alcohol comes back to you, imagine that you want to continue without alcohol only a little bit more. Never think that you will never ever drink alcohol again. Of course this would be great but for some people it is impossible to stand the idea, especially at the beginning of the therapy. But instead of breaking the abstinence right away, ALWAYS give yourself some time, even very short and say to yourself:

I will wait still one hour.

I will wait still 2 hours.

I will wait still 3 hours.

Etc.

I will wait still one day.

I will wait still 2 days.

I will wait still 3 days.

Etc.

Afer one hour or 2 hours or one day or 2 days passed by, ask yourself:

Do I feel the desire to drink alcohol?

No

In such a case you can continue with abstinence untill next time you feel the desire to drink alcohol.

Yes

In such a case you can make one more effort and one more time put untill later drinking alcohol again. Are you ready to make such an effort?

Yes

In this case you continue the abstinence.

No

In this case you are close to loose this time the battle with alcohol. This means you are not yet determined enough to continue the abstinence.

Try again later and never think when giving up drinking alcohol that it is for always. Always think it is for as long as possible.

Attention! Every time you give up alcohol you must get from your doctor drugs for the transition period between drinking alcohol and abstinence. Abrupt stop of drinking alcohol can be very dangerous for your health and even life.

***

Evening

- Repeat STOP (10 times every 2 hours).
- Say slowly every 3 hours: sun, flower, seven, path, tee, run, yellow, apple, fish, rain, pen, water, smile, talk, life, sky.
- Small supper.
- Nice talk (no complaints) 40 min. When nobody to talk with, phone or internet conversation oral or written.
- Walk 25 min.
- Every time the desire to drink alcohol comes back to you, imagine that you want to continue without alcohol only a little bit more. Never think that you will never ever drink alcohol again. Of course this would be great but for some people it is impossible to stand the idea, especially at the beginning of the therapy. But instead of breaking the abstinence right away,

ALWAYS give yourself some time, even very short and say to yourself:

I will wait still one hour.

I will wait still 2 hours.

I will wait still 3 hours.

Etc.

I will wait still one day.

I will wait still 2 days.

I will wait still 3 days.

Etc.

Afer one hour or 2 hours or one day or 2 days passed by, ask yourself:

Do I feel the desire to drink alcohol?

No

In such a case you can continue with abstinence untill next time you feel the desire to drink alcohol.

Yes

In such a case you can make one more effort and one more time put untill later drinking alcohol again. Are you ready to make such an effort?

Yes

In this case you continue the abstinence.

No

In this case you are close to loose this time the battle with alcohol. This means you are not yet determined enough to continue the abstinence. Try again later and never think when giving up drinking alcohol that it is for always. Always think it is for as long as possible.

Attention! Every time you give up alcohol you must get from your doctor drugs for the transition period between drinking alcohol and abstinence. Abrupt stop of drinking alcohol can be very dangerous for your health and even life.

***

Night

Before sleep

- Take a shower (warm water) 1 min.
- Small physical excercise 3 min.

In Bed

- Repeat STOP (20 times)
- Say slowly untill you fall asleep: sun, flower, seven, path, tee, run, yellow, apple, fish, rain, pen, water, smile, talk, life, sky.

If you cannot fall asleep

- Say slowly untill you fall asleep: sun, flower, seven, path, tee, run, yellow, apple, fish, rain, pen, water, smile, talk, life, sky.

If above does not help

- Stand up and go to the toilet (when possible with as little light as possible)
- Say slowly untill you fall asleep: sun, flower, seven, path, tee, run, yellow, apple, fish, rain, pen, water, smile, talk, life, sky.

If above does not help

- Say STOP untill you fall asleep

If above does not help

- Go to the kitchen and have a very small snack.
- Back to the bed say slowly untill you fall asleep: sun, flower, seven, path, tee, run, yellow, apple, fish, rain, pen, water, smile, talk, life, sky.

If above does not help

- Say slowly untill morning: sun, flower, seven, path, tee, run, yellow, apple, fish, rain, pen, water, smile, talk, life, sky.

***

Day 7

Morning

* Repeat STOP (10 times every 2 hours)

* Say slowly every 3 hours: sun, flower, seven, path, tee, run, yellow, apple, fish, rain, pen, water, smile, talk, life, sky.

* Small physical excercise (20 min)

* Small breakfast.

* Nice talk (no complaints) 30 min. When nobody to talk with, phone or internet conversation oral or written.

* Walk 25 min.

* Every time the desire to drink alcohol comes back to you, imagine that you want to continue without alcohol only a little bit more. Never think that you will never ever drink alcohol again. Of course this would be great but for some people it is impossible to stand the idea, especially at the beginning of the therapy. But instead of breaking the abstinence right away, ALWAYS give yourself some time, even very short and say to yourself:

I will wait still one hour.

I will wait still 2 hours.

I will wait still 3 hours.

Etc.

I will wait still one day.

I will wait still 2 days.

I will wait still 3 days.

Etc.

Afer one hour or 2 hours or one day or 2 days passed by, ask yourself:

Do I feel the desire to drink alcohol?

No

In such a case you can continue with abstinence untill next time you feel the desire to drink alcohol.

Yes

In such a case you can make one more effort and one more time put untill later drinking alcohol again. Are you ready to make such an effort?

Yes

In this case you continue the abstinence.

No

In this case you are close to loose this time the battle with alcohol. This means you are not yet determined enough to continue the abstinence.

Try again later and never think when giving up drinking alcohol that it is for always. Always think it is for as long as possible.

Attention! Every time you give up alcohol you must get from your doctor drugs for the transition period between drinking alcohol and abstinence. Abrupt stop of drinking alcohol can be very dangerous for your health and even life.

***

Afternoon

* Repeat STOP (10 times every 2 hours).

* Say slowly every 3 hours: sun, flower, seven, path, tee, run, yellow, apple, fish, rain, pen, water, smile, talk, life, sky.

* Dinner and half an hour break (you can sleep).

* Nice talk (no complaints) 40 min. When nobody to talk with, phone or internet conversation oral or written.

* Walk 25 min.

* Every time the desire to drink alcohol comes back to you, imagine that you want to continue without alcohol only a little bit more. Never think that you will never

ever drink alcohol again. Of course this would be great but for some people it is impossible to stand the idea, especially at the beginning of the therapy. But instead of breaking the abstinence right away, ALWAYS give yourself some time, even very short and say to yourself:

I will wait still one hour.

I will wait still 2 hours.

I will wait still 3 hours.

Etc.

I will wait still one day.

I will wait still 2 days.

I will wait still 3 days.

Etc.

Afer one hour or 2 hours or one day or 2 days passed by, ask yourself:

Do I feel the desire to drink alcohol?

No

In such a case you can continue with abstinence untill next time you feel the desire to drink alcohol.

Yes

In such a case you can make one more effort and one more time put untill later drinking alcohol again. Are you ready to make such an effort?

Yes

In this case you continue the abstinence.

No

In this case you are close to loose this time the battle with alcohol. This means you are not yet determined enough to continue the abstinence.

Try again later and never think when giving up drinking alcohol that it is for always. Always think it is for as long as possible.

Attention! Every time you give up alcohol you must get from your doctor drugs for the transition period between drinking alcohol and abstinence. Abrupt stop of drinking alcohol can be very dangerous for your health and even life.

***

Evening

- Repeat STOP (10 times every 2 hours).
- Say slowly every 3 hours: sun, flower, seven, path, tee, run, yellow, apple, fish, rain, pen, water, smile, talk, life, sky.

- Small supper.
- Nice talk (no complaints) 40 min. When nobody to talk with, phone or internet conversation oral or written.
- Walk 25 min.
- Every time the desire to drink alcohol comes back to you, imagine that you want to continue without alcohol only a little bit more. Never think that you will never ever drink alcohol again. Of course this would be great but for some people it is impossible to stand the idea, especially at the beginning of the therapy. But instead of breaking the abstinence right away, ALWAYS give yourself some time, even very short and say to yourself:

I will wait still one hour.

I will wait still 2 hours.

I will wait still 3 hours.

Etc.

I will wait still one day.

I will wait still 2 days.

I will wait still 3 days.

Etc.

Afer one hour or 2 hours or one day or 2 days passed by, ask yourself:

Do I feel the desire to drink alcohol?

No

In such a case you can continue with abstinence untill next time you feel the desire to drink alcohol.

Yes

In such a case you can make one more effort and one more time put untill later drinking alcohol again. Are you ready to make such an effort?

Yes

In this case you continue the abstinence.

No

In this case you are close to loose this time the battle with alcohol. This means you are not yet determined enough to continue the abstinence. Try again later and never think when giving up drinking alcohol that it is for always. Always think it is for as long as possible.

Attention! Every time you give up alcohol you must get from your doctor drugs for the transition period between drinking alcohol and abstinence. Abrupt stop of drinking alcohol can be very dangerous for your health and even life.

***

Night

Before sleep

- Take a shower (warm water) 1 min.
- Small physical excercise 3 min.

In Bed

- Repeat STOP (20 times)
- Say slowly untill you fall asleep: sun, flower, seven, path, tee, run, yellow, apple, fish, rain, pen, water, smile, talk, life, sky.

If you cannot fall asleep

- Say slowly untill you fall asleep: sun, flower, seven, path, tee, run, yellow, apple, fish, rain, pen, water, smile, talk, life, sky.

If above does not help

- Stand up and go to the toilet (when possible with as little light as possible)
- Say slowly untill you fall asleep: sun, flower, seven, path, tee, run, yellow, apple, fish, rain, pen, water, smile, talk, life, sky.

If above does not help

- Say STOP untill you fall asleep

If above does not help

- Go to the kitchen and have a very small snack.

- Back to the bed say slowly untill you fall asleep: sun, flower, seven, path, tee, run, yellow, apple, fish, rain, pen, water, smile, talk, life, sky.

If above does not help

- Say slowly untill morning: sun, flower, seven, path, tee, run, yellow, apple, fish, rain, pen, water, smile, talk, life, sky.

***

Week four

***

Day 1

Morning

* Repeat STOP (10 times every time you become anxious)

* Say slowly every time you become anxious: sun, flower, seven, path, tee, run, yellow, apple, fish, rain, pen, water, smile, talk, life, sky.

* Small physical excercise (25 min)

* Small breakfast.

* Nice talk (no complaints) 45 min. When nobody to talk with, phone or internet conversation oral or written.

* Walk 30 min.

* Every time the desire to drink alcohol comes back to you, imagine that you want to continue without alcohol only a little bit more. Never think that you will never ever drink alcohol again. Of course this would be great but for some people it is impossible to stand the idea, especially at the beginning of the therapy. But instead of breaking the abstinence right away, ALWAYS give yourself some time, even very short and say to yourself:

I will wait still one hour.

I will wait still 2 hours.

I will wait still 3 hours.

Etc.

I will wait still one day.

I will wait still 2 days.

I will wait still 3 days.

Etc.

Afer one hour or 2 hours or one day or 2 days passed by, ask yourself:

Do I feel the desire to drink alcohol?

No

In such a case you can continue with abstinence untill next time you feel the desire to drink alcohol.

Yes

In such a case you can make one more effort and one more time put untill later drinking alcohol again. Are you ready to make such an effort?

Yes

In this case you continue the abstinence.

No

In this case you are close to loose this time the battle with alcohol. This means you are not yet determined enough to continue the abstinence.

Try again later and never think when giving up drinking alcohol that it is for always. Always think it is for as long as possible.

Attention! Every time you give up alcohol you must get from your doctor drugs for the transition period between drinking alcohol and abstinence. Abrupt stop of drinking alcohol can be very dangerous for your health and even life.

***

Afternoon

* Repeat STOP (10 times every time you are anxious)

* Say slowly every time you are anxious: sun, flower, seven, path, tee, run, yellow, apple, fish, rain, pen, water, smile, talk, life, sky.

* Dinner and half an hour break (you can sleep).

* Nice talk (no complaints) 45 min. When nobody to talk with, phone or internet conversation oral or written.

* Walk 35 min.

* Every time the desire to drink alcohol comes back to you, imagine that you want to continue without alcohol only a little bit more. Never think that you will never ever drink alcohol again. Of course this would be great but for some people it is impossible to stand the idea, especially at the beginning of the therapy. But instead of breaking the abstinence right away, ALWAYS give yourself some time, even very short and say to yourself:

I will wait still one hour.

I will wait still 2 hours.

I will wait still 3 hours.

Etc.

I will wait still one day.

I will wait still 2 days.

I will wait still 3 days.

Etc.

Afer one hour or 2 hours or one day or 2 days passed by, ask yourself:

Do I feel the desire to drink alcohol?

No

In such a case you can continue with abstinence untill next time you feel the desire to drink alcohol.

Yes

In such a case you can make one more effort and one more time put untill later drinking alcohol again. Are you ready to make such an effort?

Yes

In this case you continue the abstinence.

No

In this case you are close to loose this time the battle with alcohol. This means you are not yet determined enough to continue the abstinence.

Try again later and never think when giving up drinking alcohol that it is for always. Always think it is for as long as possible.

Attention! Every time you give up alcohol you must get from your doctor drugs for the transition period between drinking alcohol and abstinence. Abrupt stop of drinking alcohol can be very dangerous for your health and even life.

***

Evening

- Repeat STOP (10 times every time you are anxious).
- Say slowly every time you are anxious) : sun, flower, seven, path, tee, run, yellow, apple, fish, rain, pen, water, smile, talk, life, sky.
- Small supper.
- Nice talk (no complaints) 45 min. When nobody to talk with, phone or internet conversation oral or written.
- Walk 35 min.
- Every time the desire to drink alcohol comes back to you, imagine that you want to continue without alcohol only a little bit more. Never think that you will never ever drink alcohol again. Of course this would be great but for some people it is impossible to stand the idea, especially at the beginning of the therapy. But

instead of breaking the abstinence right away, ALWAYS give yourself some time, even very short and say to yourself:

I will wait still one hour.

I will wait still 2 hours.

I will wait still 3 hours.

Etc.

I will wait still one day.

I will wait still 2 days.

I will wait still 3 days.

Etc.

Afer one hour or 2 hours or one day or 2 days passed by, ask yourself:

Do I feel the desire to drink alcohol?

No

In such a case you can continue with abstinence untill next time you feel the desire to drink alcohol.

Yes

In such a case you can make one more effort and one more time put untill later drinking alcohol again. Are you ready to make such an effort?

Yes

In this case you continue the abstinence.

No

In this case you are close to loose this time the battle with alcohol. This means you are not yet determined enough to continue the abstinence. Try again later and never think when giving up drinking alcohol that it is for always. Always think it is for as long as possible.

Attention! Every time you give up alcohol you must get from your doctor drugs for the transition period between drinking alcohol and abstinence. Abrupt stop of drinking alcohol can be very dangerous for your health and even life.

***

Night

Before sleep

- Take a shower (warm water) 1 min.
- Small physical excercise 5 min.

In Bed

- Repeat STOP (20 times)
- Say slowly untill you fall asleep: sun, flower, seven, path, tee, run, yellow, apple, fish, rain, pen, water, smile, talk, life, sky.

If you cannot fall asleep

- Say slowly untill you fall asleep: sun, flower, seven, path, tee, run, yellow, apple, fish, rain, pen, water, smile, talk, life, sky.

If above does not help

- Stand up and go to the toilet (when possible with as little light as possible)
- Say slowly untill you fall asleep: sun, flower, seven, path, tee, run, yellow, apple, fish, rain, pen, water, smile, talk, life, sky.

If above does not help

- Say STOP untill you fall asleep

If above does not help

- Go to the kitchen and have a very small snack.
- Back to the bed say slowly untill you fall asleep: sun, flower, seven, path, tee, run, yellow, apple, fish, rain, pen, water, smile, talk, life, sky.

If above does not help

- Say slowly untill morning: sun, flower, seven, path, tee, run, yellow, apple, fish, rain, pen, water, smile, talk, life, sky.

Congratulations! You have made 4 weeks abstinence! Be proud of yourself! Continue step by step following this Alcohol Addiction Self Therapy AAST next month and maybe longer. Good luck!

P. W. Ariveder